Praise for Tired and Hungry No More

"As a stage 4 colon cancer survivor and a health coach, Tired and Hungry No More is on my client's recommended reading list as a complete guide that covers both how to eat better and how to feel better, plus delicious recipes."

Alma Hachey, Wellness Coach and Energy Healer

"Tired and Hungry No More is definitely not your ordinary guide to health. The steps offered in this clear and easy to follow book are what I have used for myself and my clients. I suffered a TIA- transient ischemic attack, and I went from being grossly overweight with a risk to have a stroke in my 20's, to an incredibly fit, world strength endurance champion in my 60's with the energy of a 20-year-old. This book is a must read for those who have tried and failed diet after failed diet. Tired and Hungry No More is complete with beginner exercise plans, stress management, and tasty recipes to follow a healthier diet for the rest of your longer and happier life."

Nick Delgado, Ph.D., ABAAHP, CHT, author of the *Simply Healthy Cookbook* and *Acne Be Gone for Good*, DelgadoProtocol.com

"I highly recommend Tired and Hungry No More to anyone who has tried to make healthy lifestyle changes and failed. The multi-prong approach Phyllis Ginsberg uses has practical, doable action steps to get you moving in the right direction to become healthier and happier."

Gary Williams, creator of the Quick Tap Process

"Phyllis has a passion that comes from a deep compassionate place because of the challenges she has gone through in life. You can feel it in her words and tone of voice in this book. I also love how she makes all the wisdom and knowledge she has acquired to help others available in a way that allows the reader to decide for themselves what may or may not work for them and their lifestyle. I'm sure whoever reads this book will find it helpful and supportive of living a healthier and happier life."

Emmanuel Dagher, author of the International #1 bestselling book, *Easy Breezy Prosperity*

"Tired and Hungry No More is informative, inspiring, and engaging."

Mike Robbins, author of *Bring Your Whole Self to Work* and *Focus on The Good Stuff.*

"This book is a stand out in the plethora of books focusing on creating and maintaining optimal health. From the internal mindset to external pro-active steps, Phyllis guides you with compassion and clarity on a path to optimal wellness. She has deconstructed a complex matrix of what keeps us tired and hungry to create a holistic, self-empowering approach that is refreshingly effective and actually doable. Everyone needs this book!"

Vicki Dello Joio, Author and Founder of The Way of Joy Spiritual Fitness program

"Phyllis highlights the importance of eating real, whole foods as part of her holistic approach to health and wellness in "Tired and Hungry No More." I highly recommend reading this important and timely book as a way to transform your health and bring more happiness and joy into your life!"

Kristin Zellhart, Certified Nutrition Educator

"Phyllis Ginsberg's passion for health and happiness comes through in Tired and Hungry No More. As a chiropractor, I can appreciate the value she shares, in bite-size pieces. I highly recommend this book to anyone who has a desire to improve their health."

Dr. Christina Alba, of Rivulet Chiropractic,
Lafayette, CA

"Tired and Hungry No More, by Phyllis Ginsberg, is a beautifully written step by step, no-nonsense, take immediate action book that opens the door to powerful and lasting health transformation."

Staci Joy, Holistic Public Health Nurse
Entrepreneur, Author, International Speaker,
Change Agent

Tired and Hungry No More

NOT YOUR ORDINARY GUIDE TO RECLAIMING YOUR HEALTH AND HAPPINESS

Phyllis Ginsberg

Finesse
Walnut Creek, CA

Phyllis Ginsberg/Finesse
2950 Buskirk Ave., Suite 150
Walnut Creek, CA 94597
www.phyllisginsberg.com

Book Layout ©2017 BookDesignTemplates.com

Ordering Information:
Quantity sales. Special discounts are available on quantity purchases by corporations, associations, and others. For details, contact the "Special Sales Department" at the address above.

Tired and Hungry No More/Phyllis Ginsberg —1st ed.
ISBN 978-1-7336939-2-9

Contents

An Invitation for You

I invite you to contact me with your questions, comments, progress or challenges as you put *Tired and Hungry No More* into action.

Website: www.phyllisginsberg.com

Email: phyllis@phyllisginsberg.com

Facebook: www.facebook.com/phyllis.ginsberg

Look for the *Tired and Hungry No More* Facebook Group and request to join.

Need a Keynote Speaker, or someone for Breakout Sessions, Workshops or Retreats? Contact me by email.

As you read this book and benefit from it, please consider leaving a positive review on Amazon so others may find this book and benefit as well. If there is anything you think should be changed, please email me at phyllis@phyllisginsberg.com.

Introduction

My story is a Cinderella story. I grew up under the burden of responsibility an eight-year-old child should never have – doing most of the cooking and cleaning for my family while my mom struggled with her health. To say I grew up an overly responsible child is an understatement. The arthritis and migraine headaches my mom endured began when she was 19 years old, a few years before my twin sister and I were born. My memories are filled with her sitting or lying in bed watching TV or sleeping. She ate poorly, smoked, and didn't exercise and she was overweight.

My dad was gone a lot working to provide for the family. My mom stayed home, and I could tell she was unhappy. I did everything I could to keep her calm. I would never think to wake her up unless I had a cup of coffee for her. When I was in elementary school, I got myself ready each morning; cooked my own breakfast, packed a lunch, and walked to the bus stop. As I got older, I took on more responsibilities, like making menus and grocery shopping lists, and doing the shopping. I liked doing these; it made me feel as if I was doing something useful.

Just before my mom's 37th birthday, she was diagnosed with breast cancer. She had surgery and whatever treatments were available, but ten months later, she was admitted to the hospital because the cancer had spread. I had no idea what was going on, and that she'd never come home again. Three weeks later she died. I was 15 years old and was terrified of suffering as she did and dying young from a horrible disease.

As a member of American culture, my health and well-being were impacted, just like so many of my peers, by eating the standard American diet. I was a bit overweight, and it wasn't uncommon for me to gain and then lose 10 - 15 pounds a year during my teen years. Weekend eating out sometimes caused as much as a 5-pound weight gain, then I would cut back during the week to lose the weight, only to do it again the next weekend. To this day, if I overdo it, I can quickly gain weight.

At 19, I had my first real health scare, and it kicked those fears into high gear, about following my mother's path. I had my first blood test, and it showed I had seriously high cholesterol. I remembered that my mother also had extremely high cholesterol. It felt like a confirmation of my worst fears. Facing that fear, I determined I was not going to suffer her fate. I knew my way around the kitchen and grocery store, and I had an interest in cooking. This experience set the stage for my journey to health and happiness.

It's because of the experiences I had growing up, although not fun at the time, that I have been able to acquire the knowledge and expertise to write *Tired and Hungry No More*. It hasn't always been easy. My mom couldn't be the parent I needed because of the state of her health. I was afraid for her and afraid of her. I missed out on learning to connect in healthy ways, and because of my home life, at times it was difficult to concentrate and do well in school.

As an adult, I struggled with my health for many years, and when I look back, I believe it was because of fear, chronic stress, and unresolved emotions. Ten years after my mom died, I gave birth to my first child. Anger, depression, sadness, and anxiety took over as all the grief I never dealt with showed up. I wanted to cherish my new child and be a good mother, but I was facing the worst time in my life due to all the unresolved feelings. I knew I needed to change, if not for myself, then for my daughter. I made a commitment to start therapy and heal. Therapy opened my eyes to new possibilities, and I decided to become a therapist myself.

It's important to me to get this information to people who are struggling with their health and happiness – how you DON'T take care of yourself physically and emotionally takes a toll on your body, your relationships, and your life, and it impacts your loved ones too. My story is a testament to that. People who don't feel well can be unapproachable because they are tired, in pain, and irritable. And their children can grow up with problems that no parent intentionally would put on them. I want to help stop that cycle in its tracks, so that others don't have to experience what I experienced.

Overview

Tired and Hungry No More is not your ordinary "health" book. It was written for you to experience the changes you are seeking in your health and happiness. While most health books start with what to do, and what not to do, what to eat and what not to eat, and how to set up an exercise regime, etc., this book starts with, what I have found to be, the most effective way to transform your health and life.

You've probably been able to stick with a program or diet for a short time, but ultimately fail to achieve lasting results. Why is that? Because people rely on self-control and willpower. These don't work because you only have so much restraint and drive before you revert to old habits.

When you get your brain on board first, the opportunity for successfully reaching and sustaining your goals is maximized. Otherwise, you'll struggle to achieve and maintain progress. You can't diet, exercise, or do any new behavior enough to overcome the conscious or unconscious thoughts that get in the way of your desires. That's why I've started this book with Healthy Mind.

Stress, emotions, and lifestyle primarily determine your health and happiness. Only about 10% of all illnesses come from genetics. The good news is that ***control over your well-being is in your hands.***

Please don't feel bad if you haven't been able to do what you need to do for better health and increased happiness. It's not your fault. I'm going to guide you through ways of being more congruent with your thoughts, feelings, desires, and actions. Only then, when the inner conflict is gone, will you be able to easily put into action the suggestions that appeal to you.

You don't have to know what to do yet, just be willing to look at where you are and head in the direction of where you'd like to be. This is what *Tired and Hungry No More* is all about. Allow me to guide you so that you can be ready for lasting health and happiness. It's possible for you to embrace any lifestyle changes more easily once you learn how to work with your brain rather than against it.
Are you ready to get started?

Part One of *Tired and Hungry No More* is Healthy Mind. Your conscious and unconscious thoughts are what determine whether you will make positive lasting changes. Your thoughts also determine the environment in which your genes get turned on or off, depending on the hormones that are released. Stress hormones, especially cortisol, are associated with weight gain, suppression of the immune system, and decreasing concentration and memory. **Did you know you can change your thought environment to a better one?** As you begin to shift out of survival thinking your body will feel calmer, your mind will be clearer, and it will be easier to lose weight, have a healthier body, and feel happier.

Part Two is Healthy Energy. Did you know that you can build your own "healthy energy" for a more vibrant life? Yes, you! **You can learn to release stored energy and emotions that have gotten in the way of your desires by using a simple technique** called the Emotional

Freedom Technique or EFT Tapping. It's based on tapping on some of the same meridian points that have been used for thousands of years in Chinese medicine, and it is a highly effective technique in Energy Psychology. I'll show you how!

Part Three is Healthy Sleep. If you have difficulty falling asleep or staying asleep, it could be caused by low levels of melatonin, the sleep hormone. **It's possible to improve the quality of your sleep so that you can wake up feeling rested and energized throughout the day**, while also reaping the numerous health benefits of adequate sleep. This book teaches you ways to increase your melatonin level NATURALLY, along with other proven suggestions for a better night's sleep.

Part Four is Healthy Body. Most of us take our body for granted until it lets us know it's being neglected through pain, disease, injury, and so on. Committing to take care of your body (at any age) reaps so many benefits: improved digestion, elevated mood, good energy, deeper sleep, higher immunity, the ability to maintain a healthy body weight or lose weight, and much, much more.

Part Five is Healthy Eating. *Tired and Hungry No More* has recipes but is NOT a diet book. It's a lifestyle book. It's about knowing what to eat for optimal health — the food you fuel your body with makes a difference. You'll be guided to start from where you are, what to be aware of, why to eat certain foods, and exactly how to do it with ease.

Part Six includes fifty healthy recipes. Most of the recipes in *Tired and Hungry No More* are plant-based, vegan, gluten-free, and REAL FOOD that everyone can enjoy. The recipes are simple to make and will help you avoid or overcome the diet-related diseases so many people around the world are suffering from, especially diabetes and heart disease. Eat well, get healthy!

True reclaiming of your health and happiness involves honoring you. At the end of each chapter, you will find "Take Action" suggestions to help you discover what's best for you. I recommend starting with Part One: Healthy Mind. You CAN make significant improvements to your health and happiness with just a few minor changes carried out over days, weeks, months, and years.

Tired and Hungry No More is about finding what's right for you. It's based on research, science, my work with clients, and my own experience.

I'm so glad you found this book; I know what's possible for you to have a healthier, happier, and more satisfying life. I wrote this book for you.

Love, Health & Happiness,

Phyllis Ginsberg

Part One: Healthy Mind

CHAPTER 1

Why Your Efforts Haven't Worked

Tired and Hungry No More begins with what you need to know to be congruent with your thoughts, feelings, and actions, so that you can achieve and maintain your health goals. By learning about thoughts, how survival thinking keeps you stuck, and what to do differently, it's possible to ***overcome what's getting in the way of making lasting changes.***

Your conscious and unconscious thoughts determine whether or not you will make positive lasting changes. Your thoughts, especially the ones you aren't aware of, are powerful enough to prevent you from getting started, sticking with an eating or exercise plan, or maintaining what you have achieved. If your thinking isn't in alignment with what you want, you won't be able to attain or sustain your progress. Throughout this book, you will learn what you need to know about yourself and your thoughts so that you can reclaim and maintain your health and happiness.

A major reason to cultivate a healthy mind is to shift out of survival thinking. As you do, your body will feel calmer, your mind will be clearer, and it will be easier to become healthier, lose weight, and feel happier. No longer will you feel tired or hungry for the wrong reasons.

Spend time and give thought to each section in this chapter for maximum benefit. See what you identify with. Awareness is the first step to reclaiming your health and happiness. For many people, this is the missing key to finally making positive lasting lifestyle changes.

Expectations Are Thoughts

I learned about expectations and performance by observing what happened to my daughter in kindergarten. Her teacher was new to teaching and had low expectations for her students. I watched my daughter struggle to use scissors and put on her jacket while showing no interest in reading. Fortunately, this teacher went on maternity leave partway through the year, and a more experienced substitute teacher with higher expectations took over the class. Wow! What a difference I witnessed. My daughter was doing more for herself, and as she did, her scissor skills improved, she wasn't asking for help with her jacket as much, and she was taking more of an interest in books. In fact, I spoke with other parents, and we were all happy to see our children motivated about their learning and performing significantly better.

Research shows that high expectations lead to high performance while low expectations lead to a decrease in performance.[1] If you were raised with messages of low expectations from parents, teachers, or other significant people in your life, those messages were part of your early childhood programming. AND they may still run through your thoughts like a recorded loop, holding you back from your potential and your happiness.

Expectations are thoughts, and thoughts can be changed. It's never too late to shift away from low expectations to know what is best for yourself and be able to make wise decisions and sustain healthier choices, as you learn from this book.

Are you aware of your expectations about becoming healthier or happier? Do you expect it to be easy? Or, do you expect it to be difficult, to take a long time, or that you will fail again? These negative expectations are common for someone who has struggled to implement or sustain healthy choices. Generally, unless we stop and think about them, we are not consciously aware of our expectations.

What You Think May Be More Important Than What You Eat

Your thoughts are so powerful that they create feelings that determine the actions you will or will not take. Did you know that you have about 60,000 thoughts a day and of those thoughts, 95% are the same, and 80% are negative? It's not your fault! Your brain is hardwired to be on the lookout for negative experiences for survival. This way of thinking protects you from something that isn't safe. It may not feel safe (on a conscious or unconscious level) to improve your health or happiness and function as a different person from who you are today.

Imagine taking on a new identity as a healthier or happier self. How would that change you? Your relationships? And your life? Ask yourself if it's safe for you to do, be, or have what matters most to you. Get specific. Define it, see it, feel it, and then ask if it's safe.

If you answered "No," don't panic! It's normal. It just means that there is some resistance, and you aren't ready for what you want at this moment. If you know what's holding you back, you can make some adjustments to the way you think about what doesn't feel safe. If you don't have a clue why you have resistance, try to think about past failures, what you must give up to be successful, or any new responsibilities you may not feel ready for. These are just a few thoughts that could be lurking in your subconscious, trying to protect you.

Anxiety, Depression, Fear, and Worry

It's tiring to feel anxiety, depression, and fear. Add worry to that mix, and it can be truly immobilizing. Managing heavy emotions and negative thoughts are exhausting. When you have a healthy mind, (and yes, it's possible to make the shift to a healthier mind), then your thoughts and feelings will be more congruent with your desires, and that will decrease or eliminate any resistance. Once you learn how to work with your thoughts and feelings, it will get easier.

Following are brief explanations of anxiety, depression, fear, and worry:

Anxiety

Anxiety is a thought disorder. It's a way of thinking about a situation that produces distressing feelings. When anxiety produces these feelings over time, it interferes with your daily life and health. The good news is that you have the power to change your thoughts – away from anxiety and toward calmness, clarity, and peace of mind. I can help you with that!

Depression

Depression is a lack of expression. By this, I mean that sadness, grief, anger, resentment, and loneliness are feelings that don't get expressed and resolved. There are lots of reasons why depressed people don't process their feelings, and they continue to suffer, often without reaching out for help. Sometimes the thought of feeling your feelings is so overwhelming that consciously or unconsciously they are suppressed. The World Health Organization estimates that more than 300 million people worldwide suffer from depression. It's also the world's leading cause of disability.[2]

Fear

Fear is everywhere! There's fear of speaking, fear of heights, and fear of spiders. Those, however, aren't the fears I'm referring to. We live in a fear-based society. Not only do we have our own internal fears, but we also have external fears. Internally, you may fear being judged, rejected, or not measuring up, while externally you fear your neighbor, co-worker or boss. We have become a society of people who fear each other. We tend to fear people that don't think the same as us, and who don't share the same values and beliefs.

Worry

Worry is future thinking about something that may never happen. In fact, 85% of what people worry about never happens.[3] Worry gets in the way of enjoyment by focusing on what you don't want to happen rather than what you DO want to happen. This type of thinking can produce high levels of stress and stress hormones, which have negative effects on your health.

Researchers have proven, through MRI imaging, that negative thoughts stimulate the areas of the brain that promote depression and anxiety. There is a way out of worry, however. They've also confirmed that positive thoughts set off a cascade of positive hormones throughout the body that result in feelings of calm and peace.[4] Fear and worry get in the way of clear thinking, making wise decisions, and living a healthy and happy life.

Emotions Can Take a Toll on Your Body

Emotions are physical and instinctive. They alert you to immediate danger and serve to ensure immediate survival, which is a good thing. However, emotions can take a toll on your body. Anger and fear are two emotions that signal the release of cortisol and adrenaline, which, over time, can weaken your immune system, cause a debilitating illness, and contribute to weight gain.

It's helpful to recognize your emotions – to feel them and move beyond those that don't serve you. Otherwise, they get stored in your body and turn into long-lasting feelings that keep you in a state of chronic stress.

Have you tried to lose weight, yet even with eating healthy and not overeating, it's not happening? It may be due to stress hormones. A high amount of cortisol production increases insulin levels, causing a decrease in blood sugar and cravings for sugary, fatty foods.[5]

Stress and Overwhelm

When I was growing up in the 1960s, most stores were closed on Sundays, and our cable TV had seven channels that went off the air during the night when most people slept. Today, we live in a 24/7 society with no downtime. Adults are maxed out with the responsibilities of working, earning enough money, parenting, taking care of sick or elderly family members, or dealing with their own health issues. The result – stress and overwhelm! I've had so many clients tell me they desperately need a break from it all.

Do you feel that way too? Help is on the way!

As a child, I was saddled with a caregiving role, and this was one of the biggest stressors in my life. Research suggests that when children take on caregiving roles in the family, their educational, social, and emotional health can often be seriously jeopardized.[6] **My experience led me to believe I had to do it all alone. This was my programmed survival thinking.** I now know that my conscious and unconscious thoughts are at play, and this isn't really the truth. I know it's possible to shift my thoughts and decrease my stress.

When you're stressed and overwhelmed, you tend to run on auto-pilot, lacking the ability to think clearly. Chronic stress can have an adverse effect on you physically, emotionally, and mentally. It prevents you from being available to yourself and others in the ways that you want to be but can't. Throughout this book, you will discover numerous pieces of information and practical suggestions that will help you reclaim your health and happiness. I believe it all starts with your conscious and unconscious thoughts. As you'll soon read, it is possible to shift your thoughts and decrease your stress. It's the first step, and then you will start to see the evidence of your situation improving.

The Brain Doesn't Know the Difference

A fascinating fact about the brain is this: It doesn't know if you actually DID something or just thought about it! So, when you have pleasant, calm, or happy thoughts, your brain believes something wonderful has happened and signals the release of the "feel good" hormones serotonin and dopamine. When you have anxious, negative thoughts, your brain signals the release of the "stress hormones" cortisol and adrenaline.

How you think has a direct effect on how you feel. Since your thoughts produce either healthy or unhealthy chemical releases into your body, then this means you have some control over your well-being.[7] What great news!

Now, don't micromanage your thoughts – that produces its own set of anxiety and stress! Just become aware of the thoughts you have, acknowledge them ("good" or "bad"), and then replace them with new thoughts that will result in greater well-being. You'll learn how to do this in the first two parts of this book.

Why choose thoughts that support a healthy mind? You think more clearly, make better decisions, are more focused, sleep better, feel calmer, face difficulties with greater ease, and, of course, feel happier!

What If I Don't Know My Thoughts?

Most of us don't know what our thoughts are because 95% of them occur outside of our awareness. How, then, can you know whether or not your thoughts are healthy for you? One clue is to notice how you feel. Are you feeling angry? It might be that you're thinking, "It's not fair!" "How dare they treat me like that?" Or, "I don't WANT to."

When you're feeling sad, you might be thinking, "I don't want to suffer like this." "I wish I could be like everybody else." Or, "I miss my _____." (Fill in the blank with something or someone you don't have anymore.)

Take some time to practice noticing how you feel, and what you might be thinking to cause that feeling. And be patient with yourself, as it's common not to be consciously aware of your thoughts or feelings – that's the way the human brain was designed, to protect us from too much stimuli. The way I started becoming aware of my feelings and thoughts was to ask myself a few times a day, "what am I feeling? and "what am I thinking?" I used a timer to remind me to check in with myself and made Post-it notes with the two questions. With practice, you'll get better at becoming aware of your feelings and thoughts, and then have more control over your thinking so that you can let those thoughts roll through you, rather than control your moods.

Are You Afraid of Your Feelings?

It's a cultural norm to avoid feelings. Many people try to numb their uncomfortable feelings with food, shopping, spending money, watching TV, excess time on social media and other unproductive ways. It can be overwhelming to feel strong emotions. But the truth is that the more we avoid them, the more they show up in our moods and our bodies, whether or not we're aware of it.

The number one reason I hear from people about suppressing their emotions is the fear that their emotions will be out of control, and they won't be able to function. Also, I think this fear is enhanced by the fact that when we stuff our emotions, we keep the pressure on until they implode out of control. The urgency to act is much greater because the pressure is greater. I'm going to teach you how to face and embrace your feelings, so they don't show up as stress, worry, anxiety, or depression.

Why Do We Self-Medicate with Food?

When we don't want to feel bad, food is an effective and easy way to feel better. Certain foods provide a "feel good" response in the brain, so we may keep eating those foods even though they aren't nourishing our bodies. And the feeling is temporary, so we "need" more, thus overeating, eating too much comfort food (carbs and sugar), and binge eating. More than ever before, adults and children are abusing their bodies with food in order to not feel or to fill a void, which creates food-related illnesses. Then they rely on medication to manage their symptoms and diseases, and the cycle continues.

It CAN be different. If you are one of the millions of people who struggle with one or more of the following: diabetes, high blood pressure, high cholesterol, high triglycerides, heart disease, acid reflux, chronic pain, or sleep apnea, this book may change your life! If you currently have or had cancer or a stroke in the past, it may not be too late to give your body its best chance of recovering.

My Near Burnout

Let's talk about BURNOUT... In 2005, I was working 12 - 14 hours a day in private practice on court-appointed cases dealing with high conflict divorce. While I loved the work and was great at it, I lost me. I was trying to do everything for everybody else and forgot to include me! I suffered from burnout. My health declined, and I knew I had to do something different.

I grew up doing what I thought I was supposed to do, and I was living that out, again. I didn't know it, but I was in survival mode and wasn't paying attention to the amount of stress I was under. I took on way too much work. It wasn't humanly possible to have any balance in my life, my work, or my relationships. I tried to do it all; be a good wife, mother, and therapist.

A big "aha" moment was when I stopped and realized that my life wasn't working for me. I woke up one morning and started thinking about what I was missing out on. While I was helping children and families cope with their difficult situations, I was missing out on spending quality time with my children and husband. I was also missing me – the me that was healthy and vibrant. I was exhausted all the time as I did what I learned to do so well growing up – put on a happy face and make sure everyone else is okay.

This was the first time I honestly knew I couldn't continue putting everyone else first while neglecting myself and feeling neglected by others, because I didn't share how bad I was feeling with anyone.

I took some time off and immersed myself in the field of Positive Psychology. Every day that I focused on applying what I discovered from brain research, I got myself back in a way I had not ever felt before. I became happy. ***The cloud of grief that loomed over me for two decades had lifted.*** My health improved, and so did my relationships!

Now, I help others do the same. I know what's possible for you because it was possible for me. It doesn't have to be difficult or take a long time to see, feel, and experience improved health and increased happiness.

Why Happiness?

A reasonable question, especially in a society where so many people try to "buy" happiness and find that it doesn't work – they're still stressed, anxious, can't sleep, have health issues, and even feel chronically depressed.

Let's turn to the relatively new field of Positive Psychology for some answers about why happiness is healthy. Studies show that people who are happy have better health. One reason is that people who are happier are less stressed. You can't experience high levels of stress and be genuinely happy at the same time.

Here's the key: It's not about what you "have," it's the frequent experience and expression of positive emotions that create resilience and resourcefulness.[8] These traits make it easier to get through life, connect with others, and take good care of yourself. A healthy mind allows for a greater ability to solve problems, come up with good ideas, and to get through life with greater ease. Do these sound like happiness-making traits? Yes!

That doesn't mean that happy people don't ever feel fear, anger, or sadness. What makes them different is the ability to sense feelings and not get stuck in them. People who are happier aren't weighed down with problems. They aren't plagued with worry, lack of sleep, and negativity. They have the energy, stamina, and vitality to get through each day and they course correct when necessary. Happy people go about life with excitement and passion. They wake up every day ready to see what will happen. Overall, they feel satisfied with their life.

Something as simple as a happy thought, smiling, or laughing can shift your emotions from negative to positive. Over time, the experience and expression of positive emotions will become more automatic.

Have You Made a Resolution, a Declaration, or a Commitment?

So, you want to get healthy or become happier? Have you made a resolution, like a New Year's resolution? Have you declared to yourself or to someone else that you are going to make some changes? It's going to take more than a simple resolution or declaration to create a long-term healthy lifestyle, but it's necessary because you must do something different, on purpose, if you want a different result. It's going to take committing yourself.

The human brain does best with small changes, building new neural pathways as you experience a series of mini-successes, which grow into healthy, happy habits and big, long-lasting results. Try committing to a small change and see what happens.

For example:

- You might commit to reading or thinking about something that makes you feel happy, calm, and relaxed 15 minutes before turning out the lights to go to sleep.

- You may want to commit to moving your body by getting up every hour to stretch or walk around a bit, so you don't end up sitting for hours at work, at home, or in the car.

- Or, you could commit to starting your day with a healthy, nutritious breakfast. Did you know that when you start your day with a healthy meal, you're more likely to continue eating well your next meal? So, try committing to starting your day with a healthy, nutritious breakfast. Start small by planning what you will have the night before, so you don't leave it up to chance when you are hungry that you will make a healthy choice.

You Are What You Eat – Is Not Exactly True!

Of course, you're going to read and learn some great things about eating healthy in this book, along with some delicious recipes to support you. But let's go a little deeper than food...

What if unresolved thoughts, feelings, and experiences are what drive you to make the choices you make about your body? Such as:

- What you feed your body
- How much you feed it
- If you exercise it
- Whether you treat your body as a friend or foe

All of these outcomes are driven by experiences we've had throughout our lives that have been painful, fearful, and heavy with emotion. You may have experienced a significant illness, injury, loss, financial hardship, relationship or family conflict, work, or career-related challenge.

What's weighing you down? What experiences from your life, past or present, feel heavy? What burdens are you carrying around? What's weighing you down and preventing you from traveling with ease in a lighter healthier body? Take some time to answer these questions. By becoming aware of what's going on inside of you, it's possible to feel some relief from the thoughts and feelings that are weighing heavily on you.

Care or Curse Your Body?

On a continuum, of lovingly caring for your body on one end, and cursing your body on the other, where do you see yourself and your relationship to your body? Do you feel let down, betrayed, or embarrassed by your body? Do you appreciate all that your body does for you? Your thoughts about your body impact how it functions and how you treat it.

You only get one body, and the messages you tell yourself about your body can significantly affect how well you care for yourself. What if treating your body with kindness was the answer to feeling better, less stressed, more confident, and possibly the solution to overcoming an illness, injury, or weight issue?

Consider treating your body with love, care, kindness, and the respect you and your body deserve using the following five steps.

Five Steps to Treating Your Body with Kindness

1. Define what treating your body with kindness is for you. It could be one of these or something else.

- Getting more sleep or rest
- Eating better
- Exercising or some other movement
- Appreciating your body

2. Notice your self-talk about your body when you say:

- I can't…
- I don't want to…
- I'm not ready to…

3. Plan what you will do differently. (You MUST do something different from what you are doing now.)

- What will you do to get more sleep, eat better, move your body, or appreciate your body?
- Think small. One tiny change in the right direction will get you closer to treating your body with more kindness than doing nothing.

- Calendar it! Yes, decide and commit to treating your body with kindness by scheduling it in your calendar as an appointment.

4. Expect a positive outcome as you carry out your plan of doing something small to treat your body with kindness.

5. Celebrate!

- Acknowledge your small win.
- Share it with a friend.
- Post it in the *Tired and Hungry No More* Facebook group.
- Give yourself a pat on the back! Tell yourself, "I did it!"

These acts of celebration will anchor in your accomplishment.

Small wins over time lead to significant results!

Best Friend or Worst Enemy?

You can be your own best friend or worst enemy. Most of us would never speak to a friend the way we talk to ourselves. It's common for people to be harder on themselves than anyone else. This ingrained automatic thinking comes from an inner critic that can interfere with your efforts to be happy and healthy, to have satisfying relationships, or to reach your work or financial goals.

Notice when you are judging yourself harshly. Stop and acknowledge the thought. When you acknowledge your thoughts, they have less power over you. It's like saying, "I see you, and I'm on to you."

You can become your own best friend by talking to yourself in ways that you would to someone you genuinely cared about or to a trusted friend.

Take Action:

When you see something in this book that you'd like to do or try, take some action right away; within 24 hours is ideal. You'll be more likely to do it before you forget, lose interest, or talk yourself out of it. When you tell yourself you'll get back to it, realistically, you never will.

As humans, much of what we think about is out of our awareness and negative. That's how we were designed, for survival. It has served us well, AND there is a better way. Positive Psychology has paved the way for happiness, better health, more resiliency, and closer connections.

Do one or more of the following to reclaim your health and happiness:

1. Replace thoughts of fear and worry with pleasant, calm, or happy thoughts. Remember, your brain doesn't know if you did something or just thought about it.

2. Think about something that makes you happy, brings you joy, or that you feel grateful for. Do this when you wake up in the morning or just before falling asleep at night.

3. Set aside some time to become aware of your expectations. Write down any thoughts you have, positive or negative, about

something you want. Then ask yourself, "What would I be thinking if I expected a positive outcome?" See if you can imagine yourself expecting something wonderful to happen.

4. Increase your happiness by smiling and laughing with others. This will produce feel good hormones.

5. Notice when you have negative thoughts about yourself or your body and replace them with thoughts that speak more highly of YOU!

6. Make a commitment to yourself to do one small thing to become healthier and happier.

7. Use the Five Steps to Treating Your Body with Kindness (on page 16).

8. Answer the following questions from the section, "You Are What You Eat – Is Not Exactly True!" It may give you clues to what's unresolved.

❖ What experiences from your life, past or present, feel heavy?

❖ What burdens are you carrying around?

❖ What's weighing you down and preventing you from traveling with ease in a lighter, healthier body?

Notes

[1] Self-Fulfilling Prophecy in Psychology
https://positivepsychologyprogram.com/self-fulfilling-prophecy/

[2] Depression: Facts, Statistics, and You
https://www.healthline.com/health/depression/facts-statistics-infographic#1

[3] 85% of What We Worry About Never Happens
https://donjosephgoewey.com/eighty-five-percent-of-worries-never-happen-2/

[4] Don't Believe Everything You Think
http://www.clevelandclinicwellness.com/programs/NewSFN/pages/default.aspx?Lesson=3&Topic=2&UserId=00000000-0000-0000-0000-000000000705

[5] Stress and Weight Gain
https://www.webmd.com/diet/features/stress-weight-gain#1

[6] The Impact of Parental Illness and Disability on Children's Caring Roles
https://onlinelibrary.wiley.com/doi/pdf/10.1111/1467-6427.00121

[7] Health Benefits of a Healthy Mind
https://www.mayoclinic.org/healthy-lifestyle/stress-management/in-depth/positive-thinking/art-20043950

---

[8] Positive Emotions and Wellbeing
https://www.psychologytoday.com/blog/between-cultures/201611/positive-emotions-and-wellbeing

CHAPTER 2

Where Are You In Your Life?

I've had a skewed relationship with time. For a good part of my life, my time was not my own. I learned to cook and clean at the age of eight to fill in for my mother who couldn't physically do much due to her chronic pain. As a result, I became an over-responsible child who was on hyper-alert, to make sure my parents were okay so that I felt safe.

As a grownup, I also spent most of my time putting others first. I can remember numerous times as a mother when I suddenly had some time to myself, unable to decide what to do. Having time to myself felt so foreign to me. I wasn't used to putting myself first or acknowledging that I had needs. Have you ever had that experience?

Perhaps you experienced getting to the point of exhaustion, irritability, and resentment. "Why does it feel like I'm there for everybody else?" "Why can't so-and-so do this herself?" "When do I get to live my life?" And even: "Why BE here if I exist to make everyone else's life easier?"

Here's the thing: You can only function for so long without recharging yourself with adequate sleep and activities that sustain you. When all your energy goes out and very little comes back, you're headed for a health crisis.

If you think you don't have time to do something for yourself, think again. It's VITAL for your health and happiness that you carve out some time for yourself to do things that sustain you, are meaningful to you, and bring you joy.

Yeah, Yeah, I Know You're Busy...

Are you going to wait until you're sick to give yourself a break? Your mind and body can handle a lot, but at what price? Without some leisure time, you can't slow down enough to listen to your thoughts, your body, and your intuition.

So where can you fit 30 minutes into your day for self-care? Try self-care first thing in the morning, before work, during a lunch break, after work, before dinner, while the kids are at sports practice, doing homework or doing another activity, after dinner, or before bed. Experiment with different times until you find a time slot that works for you.

Start today! Slow down and incorporate some leisure into your day. Go for an enjoyable walk, hike, swim or bike ride, work on a craft, read a book or magazine, drive at the pace of other cars rather than passing them, or do any other activity for the pure enjoyment of it.

Did you know that 30 minutes is just 2% of a 24-hour day? You are worth the time! Creating a healthy lifestyle and a healthy body may take less time than you think. Research shows that just 30 minutes of daily movement, like walking, is enough to make a positive difference in your health.[1] It doesn't matter what you do with your time as long as it's beneficial to you. It could be doing something physical, something relaxing, or something creative.

Is It Time to Ask for Help?

It's not my intention to suggest there is something seriously "wrong" with you and you'd better do something about it. For so many of us, asking for help is very difficult. There are so many good reasons to ask for help, delegate, or hire someone. It's also possible to figure out other ways to accomplish goals by working with others. Carpools, co-working, or masterminding, and finding a walking buddy are good examples.

Working with others offers us a new experience, new ideas, and new ways of doing things we would never have thought of. We get inspired, motivated, and held accountable to do things that are good for us.

An increasing number of Americans say they often or always feel alone. Loneliness is a growing health epidemic according to former Surgeon General Doctor Vivek Murthy. Asking for help, making connections, and being with others is, in fact, healthy for you!

A 2018 survey of more than 20,000 U.S. adults 18 years and older showed the following:

- More than half reported sometimes or always feeling alone (46%) or left out (47%). Forty-three percent sometimes or always feel that their relationships are not meaningful, and they are isolated from others.

- Americans who live with others are less likely to be lonely (average loneliness score of 43.5) compared to those who live alone (46.4). However, this does not apply to single parents/guardians (average loneliness score of 48.2) even though they live with children; they are more likely to be lonely.

- Only around half of Americans (53%) have meaningful in-person social interactions, such as having an extended conversation with a friend or spending quality time with family, on a daily basis.

- Those between ages 18-22 were the loneliest group, feeling alone or lacking social connectedness, and claimed to be in worse health than older generations.[2]

Isolation is another risk factor for poor health:

- More than 8 million adults age 50 and older are affected by isolation, which is different from loneliness. Isolation is when someone is physically or emotionally disconnected from friends, family, and community. Prolonged isolation is increasingly recognized as a risk factor for poor health.[3]

In the next section, you'll read about support and connection, the antidote to loneliness and isolation.

Support and Connection

Many of us appear to be doing well on the outside, when the truth is, we are not doing well on the inside. Can you relate? My mom wasn't emotionally or physically available most of the time while I was growing up, so I spent a great deal of my childhood feeling alone and isolated. After her death, (when I was only 15), my peers didn't know how to relate to me, and I didn't know how to seek out help or support to deal with my grief. I endured life's challenges alone. It's typical for girls who grow up with a chronically ill parent to adopt caregiving tasks, and they tend to be at higher risk for stress, depressive symptoms, and other internalized problem behaviors.[4] This was my template, and it is still something I continue to work on.

Throughout my life, even when I didn't feel well, I still functioned as a mom, a wife, and a professional at work. It wasn't until 2005 when I suffered from near burnout in every area of my life that I decided to take some time off, and once again reconnect with myself.

I learned that emotional support often came from friends who didn't share my history, rather than from family. Friends were more willing to listen and offer different perspectives because they were more objective and less invested.

As I connected more with myself through keeping a "Happiness Journal" at night and doing daily meditation in the morning, my thoughts began to change. I felt more relaxed, and I had increased energy. It became easier to stay connected to myself and with others. I made a point to get together with friends. We walked, we talked, and sometimes we would cook together. I felt happy engaging in mutual conversation, which was something I couldn't do with clients. I hadn't realized how socially deprived I felt until I stopped working and began connecting with friends. Connection with others is a positive, healthy factor to longevity.

However, many of us, especially women, don't want to bother or burden others. We don't ask for help or support. Meanwhile, the people close to us aren't aware that we are suffering.

Two things need to happen for you to get support and connection. First, you have to ask for what you need or seek it out. Second, you must be willing to receive it. It's not weak to ask for help, see a therapist, or hire a coach. Through my healing from burnout, I learned to become more vulnerable and see vulnerability as a strength, not a weakness. Showing vulnerability relieves our true self, which attracts the people who can understand our problems and concerns and offer support.[5]

What Are You Looking Forward To?

No matter what your age, having something to look forward to that's fun, special, or different can help you get through your day-to-day routine. The anticipation of an upcoming event, outing, or get-together builds excitement and may even cause you to daydream about it, giving you a positive experience similar to being in meditation.

When you have something to look forward to you may experience yourself smiling more, being kinder to others and yourself, and more tolerant of things that generally annoy you. In other words, having something to look forward to may have a positive effect on your happiness, well-being, and even your productivity.

What are you looking forward to?[6]

Take Action:

If your days are packed with too much to do, it may be time to evaluate how you are spending your time. This is YOUR life, and if you're not feeling satisfied, excited, or inspired, it's time to do something different. Time is your greatest currency. Once it's gone, you can't get it back.

Make time for what matters most by doing one or more of the suggestions below:

1. Find, and calendar, a 30-minute time slot each day for you to do something that sustains you. It could be anything that you enjoy or that makes you feel healthier or happier.

2. Figure out a new way of doing something to free up more time. Delegate, collaborate, coordinate, or hire someone.

3. Make a list of things you can look forward to daily, weekly, or monthly. Plan something for tomorrow, this week, this month, this year and beyond. Get out your calendar and schedule several things to look forward to.

Notes

[1] Fitness Benefits of Walking Every Day
https://www.prevention.com/fitness/benefits-walking-every-day

[2] Cigna U.S. Loneliness Survey
https://www.multivu.com/players/English/8294451-cigna-us-loneliness-survey/

[3] The Growing Impact of Isolation - AARP Bulletin July/August 2018

[4] Problem Behavior in Children of Chronically Ill Parents
https://www.ncbi.nlm.nih.gov/pmc/articles/PMC2975921

[5] Six Powerful Benefits of Vulnerability and Shame
https://intentioninspired.com/6-powerful-benefits-of-vulnerability-and-shame/

[6] *Brain Makeover – A Weekly Guide to a Happier, Healthier and More Abundant Life*, Phyllis Ginsberg (Walnut Creek: Finesse, 2014)

CHAPTER 3

Reaching Your Full Potential

If a plant gets too much water or sunlight it dies or doesn't grow to its full potential. If a human overeats food on a regular basis, they also don't develop to their full potential, creating physical disease and a poor self-image, which can affect all areas of life from relationships to work.

For us humans, the effects of overeating generally are not immediate. The first evidence of overeating is usually weight gain, that tends to "creep up" on us. It can take decades for illness to set in. Many people are not aware of having high cholesterol, high triglycerides, high blood pressure, or heart disease, because symptoms are not recognizable until they become severe enough.

Being mindful of both what and how much you eat and drink is the first step to awareness, regardless of whether you want to or are ready to make any changes.

Are You Ready?

Are you ready to see yourself differently? This is an important thing to think about! If you have an image of yourself as being unhealthy, out of shape, or unhappy and you can't imagine yourself any different, it will get in the way of making progress.

What happens when you desire to become healthier, yet your identity has been as an unhealthy person. Or, when you want to lose a significant amount of weight, and your identity has been as an overweight person? You have an internal conflict. The difference between how you are today and how you'd like to be might feel like a big gap and really hard to imagine. But it's possible - in fact, necessary, in order for you to become that person!

The person you are today is not the same person you will be when you are slim, fit, healthy, happier, or any other way you'd like to become. That's how powerful our thoughts and imagination are. Now that I have brought this to your awareness, are you ready to see yourself as slim, fit, healthy, happier? You don't have to be able to see it yet. You just need to be willing and open to it.

Enjoy What You Eat

Do you have certain foods you really like, even though they may not be the healthiest? If you don't want to give them up, there is a method to keep you from overeating them. Mindfulness is the act of paying close attention to what you are doing. By applying mindfulness to eating, you slow down the process.

Try this mindfulness exercise:

1. Take your first bite, a forkful or spoonful of food.
2. Smell the food as it enters your mouth.
3. Savor it in your mouth before you chew and swallow it.
4. Feel the texture on your tongue.
5. Chew it slowly and thoroughly before swallowing.

Now, before taking another bite, ask yourself if the first one was delicious. Rate it on a scale of 1 - 3.

1 = No, it was okay, not very satisfying and not worth the calories.
2 = No, it was good but not great.
3 = Yes, it was delicious, and worth every calorie!

Then, based on your rating, ask yourself if it would feel good to have another bite. If so, then repeat the same mindfulness approach with the second bite. Mindfully taste the food, savor it, and chew it slowly and thoroughly. Then rate that bite. Ask yourself if you would like another bite. Continue to do this until you reach a point where you don't desire more. Usually the first, second, and maybe the third bites of anything are the best, and after that you eat what is in front of you, not thinking about if the food is satisfying to you any longer.

Enjoy what you eat, one bite at a time!

Would You Like to Be More Self-Disciplined?

Have you ever said, "I shouldn't eat that second piece of [fill in the blank] ...well, just this once..." Then you feel guilty afterward for eating it? Or you say, "I really need to get this work project done today since it's due tomorrow morning!" Then you get distracted, never work on it, and feel stressed because you have to get up extra early the next morning to complete the project on time.

These situations deplete our energy, raise our anxiety, and take a toll on our feelings about ourselves as trustworthy and worthy people. How do we learn self-discipline? While self-discipline is more natural for some and more difficult for others, it comes down to finding the willingness to take small steps in the direction of your goals, ***even when you don't feel like it.*** I suggest you identify an area you'd like to improve and then decide what small steps you can begin to do toward that goal. It's wise to make no more than one or two small changes until you've mastered them, and they become a habit.

It may be helpful to visually track your progress by using a check-off chart. You can download one by visiting my website.

Track your progress with your own Check-Off Chart.
Download it at
www.phyllisginsberg.com/resources

New Habits Take More Than 21 Days

A study published in the *European Journal of Social Psychology* determined that on average, it takes more than two months before a new behavior becomes automatic — 66 days to be exact. How long it takes a new habit to form can vary widely depending on the behavior, the person, and the circumstances. In the study, it took anywhere from 18 days to 254 days for people to form a new habit.

Know that new habits take more than 21 days to become embedded and automatic. So, set your expectations appropriately. The truth is that it will probably take you anywhere from two months to eight months to build a new behavior into your life — not 21 days. Interestingly, the researchers also found that you don't have to be perfect. Missing one opportunity to perform the behavior did not materially affect the habit formation process. In other words, it doesn't matter if you mess up now and then.

Building better habits is not an all-or-nothing process. Understanding this from the beginning makes it easier to manage your expectations and commit to making small incremental improvements rather than pressuring yourself into thinking that you must do it all at once.[1]

Monitor Your Course

When traveling by car, boat, airplane, or spacecraft, the driver or pilot must monitor the course and make adjustments as necessary. You can apply this same principle to your body, your health, and your weight.

When you pay attention to how your body feels, you can tell when you are hungry, tired, or rundown. These signals cue you to eat, get some rest or sleep, and take better care of yourself.

If you are interested in decreasing your body weight or maintaining a specific weight, it's helpful to monitor how you are doing by weighing yourself every day or two. Use a scale as a tool to give you information. Please don't obsess about your weight. The information you get will inform you about your progress and when to adjust your eating or physical activity. Avoiding the scale is a decision that makes us more fearful, not less. To know exactly where we are is helpful, which is better than feeling helpless because we don't want to know.

Running on Empty

Do those you care about get the best of you or what's left of you? Do they get the crumbs of energy leftover from a difficult night or stressful day? How often do you push yourself when you are running on empty?

Our vehicles have gauges, and if we pay attention, so do our bodies. If you don't override your feelings, you can tune into when you are hungry, tired, or mentally fatigued. It is sad but true that people often take better care of their cars than they do of themselves. So today, take a short break when you need to, fuel your body with healthy foods and water so it can function optimally, and take a nap or get some sleep when you feel tired.

---

7 Quick and Easy Ways to Recharge Your Battery

Wouldn't you enjoy having good energy throughout your day? While these tips aren't a substitute for a sound night's sleep, these will help you recharge WITHOUT relying on consuming food and drinks with caffeine, sugar, and simple carbohydrates to make it through:

- Meditate for 20 minutes.
- Take a 20 - 30-minute nap.
- Go for a 10 - 20-minute walk, stretch, or do yoga.

- Drink a big glass of water.
- Listen to enjoyable music.
- Eat a piece of fruit.
- Take a bath.

A Breathing Meditation

Breathing is one way to calm your nervous system, reduce stress, and restore clearer thinking. Meditation or breathing exercises that include slow deep breaths are like putting on an oxygen mask.

Breathing is a bodily function that is both automatic and controllable. The focus of this meditation is on allowing your body to breathe itself.

Here's how to do it:

1. Get into a comfortable position, either sitting up or laying down.

2. Take several slow deep breaths to calm your body.

3. Once relaxed, slow your breathing down even more, so that you are taking fewer breaths per minute.

4. Next, let your breath happen on its own without you starting it. You'll feel when you need to take your next breath.

5. Continue this slow body breathing for up to 20 minutes.

6. Take a couple of minutes to come out of this breathing meditation. Gently begin to move your fingers and toes, then your hands and feet, and finally, your arms and legs, to bring you out of the deep relaxation.

7. Notice when your breathing has increased to a more normal pace. Then get up slowly.

Don't be surprised if you feel like you just slept for a couple of hours. While sleep is essential, an extremely relaxed meditation experience can be equivalent to several hours of sleep.

Take Action:

This chapter introduced several ways to become aware of what you need to be at your best and what to do. It first starts with your self-image, your habits, and how willing you are to make some small changes.

When you are aware of how your body feels you can do what it takes to give it what it needs and reach your full potential. Experiment with one or more of the following suggestions:

1. Imagine yourself, if you can, being the person you'd like to become.

2. Enjoy what you eat. Use mindfulness eating, especially with your favorite, not so healthy foods.

3. Notice when you are hungry and when you are full. Eat when you are hungry and stop eating when you feel full.

4. Become self-disciplined. Be willing to take small steps in the direction of your goals, even when you don't feel like it. Download and print the Check-Off Chart to track your progress. Go to www.phyllisginsberg.com/resources.

5. Monitor your progress if you desire to lose or maintain weight. Weigh yourself every day or two and "course correct" as needed.

6. Get adequate sleep, and when you don't, use some of the suggestions from this chapter to recharge.

7. Try the breathing meditation (on page 37).

Notes

[1] How Long Does it Actually Take to Form a New Habit?
https://jamesclear.com/new-habit

Part Two: Healthy Energy

CHAPTER 4

The Next Big Frontier: Energy Healing

I've known about Energy Healing from the time I was 20 years old when I took a course on kinesiology. Energy Medicine, and Energy Psychology are based on centuries old, proven methods developed using the energy systems of the body. Acupuncture and acupressure are two popular forms. Research and brain scans have provided evidence of their effectiveness in healing. The scientific evidence for Energy Psychology, Energy Medicine and Energy Healing keep growing, and millions of people experience life-changing results from these practices.[1]

The Emotional Freedom Technique

My special expertise is the "Emotional Freedom Technique" (EFT Tapping), and you'll learn how to do it in this book, with specific training, techniques, charts, and scripts to use so you can use it for yourself. It's the most effective modality I know to quickly, safely, and permanently provide relief of stress, anxiety, and unhealthy emotions. I had the privilege of knowing Dr. Roger Callahan, who developed Thought Field Therapy and who pioneered tapping on meridian points, used in Chinese medicine. I used his method of tapping to decrease my anxiety before taking the oral exam to get licensed as a therapist. To put it in perspective, the oral exam was more anxiety provoking to me than childbirth!

Dr. Callahan's work was later simplified by Gary Craig and became known as EFT Tapping. EFT Tapping is used to release blocked energy and works for anxiety, fears, phobias, stress, and for some people, it reduces physical pain. Brain scans have shown that EFT Tapping calms the amygdala, the part of the brain that responds to stress and signals the fight or flight response by producing stress hormones.[2] Stress hormones, cortisol, and adrenaline have been shown to cause weight gain and have a negative impact on the immune system.

EFT Tapping:

- Frees the energy flow throughout the meridians in your body.
- As the name says, the Emotional Freedom Technique frees stored emotions in your body.
- Rewires the brain, creating new neural pathways.

EFT Tapping can be effective without any specialized training. Here's how it works: You will be doing tapping on meridian points on your face and body. All you need to do is take two fingers and tap lightly on each of the tapping points as you say some statements. It's that easy. If you're new to EFT Tapping, you can watch an introduction to tapping video, on my website.

https://www.phyllisginsberg.com/tapping-with-phyllis.

I invite you to experience EFT Tapping by using the Tapping Points chart below. Now would be a great time to do a round of tapping, without any statements, to get familiar with the feel of it.

Take two fingers and tap lightly several times on the Eyebrow Point, where your eyebrow starts closest to your nose on either side of your face. Then tap on the Side of the Eye Point (on the bone near the eye). Next, tap several times Under Your Eye, (on the bone just under the pupil of your eye). Then tap Under Your Nose. Next, tap in the Chin crease. Then on the Collarbone, (tap on one side or the other). Move to Under Arm, tap about 4 inches from your armpit. And the last tapping point is Top of Head.

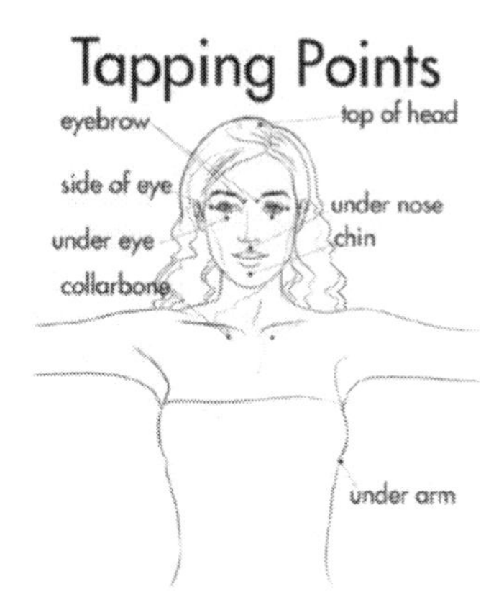

Tapping Points Abbreviations:

EB (eyebrow)
SE (side of eye)
UE (under eye)
UN (under nose)
CH (chin)
CB (collarbone)
UA (under the arm)
TH (top of head)

Take Action:

The Emotional Freedom Technique is the most effective modality I know of to quickly, safely, and permanently provide relief of stress, anxiety, and emotions.

Familiarize yourself with the tapping points and abbreviations so you will be ready to use the tapping scripts in the next chapter.

1. Study the tapping points chart and the order of the tapping points.

2. Do a round of tapping to get the feel of it.

3. Watch the video demonstration of EFT Tapping on my website at https://www.phyllisginsberg.com/tapping-with-phyllis

Notes

[1] The Science Behind Energy Psychology
https://cdn.ymaws.com/www.energypsych.org/resource/resmgr/research/Science_Behind_EP_Quick_Fact.pdf

[2] EFT Tapping Research
http://www.eftuniverse.com/research-studies/eft-research

https://www.thetappingsolution.com/science-and-research

https://www.huffingtonpost.com/entry/comprehensive-research-analysis-shows-eft-emotional_us_58868d51e4b08f5134b623da

CHAPTER 5

EFT Tapping with Tapping Scripts

In the previous chapter you learned what the Emotional Freedom Technique is and the tapping points. In this chapter, you will be tapping on specific topics with statements I have included. Each of the ten tapping scripts has three rounds of tapping for the most impact.

Round One

The first round is to acknowledge a thought or a feeling. You can do this first round several times until you feel a reduction of the intensity of the thought or feeling. Feel free to modify any of the statements to feel truer to you.

Round Two

The second round of tapping introduces possibilities. When possibilities are introduced, it gives your brain a new channel to function from. Rather than focusing on a problem, you will be guided to several options. The introduction of possible solutions serves two purposes: One is that you may like one of the solutions, the other, and more important, is that you begin to grow new neural pathways in your brain as you become solution focused.

Round Three

The third round of tapping is anchoring. This round anchors in a positive outcome or state of being. Most people feel good as they tap and say the anchoring statements, although it is not uncommon, if you are not ready for them, to feel more stress. It's not your fault. Remember, 95% of your thoughts are out of your awareness and resistance is normal. We are creatures of habit, and you may not be ready to shift something just yet. Or, it could be that you need to go back and acknowledge a thought or a feeling. The clearer you are about your thoughts and feelings, the more effective the tapping will be.

Added Tips for Best Results

Don't rush the process. When you do Tapping on one topic, another related one may show up. It doesn't mean the tapping isn't working; it just means that you got in touch with something else to acknowledge with tapping. You may become aware of subconscious thoughts that have been driving a behavior, keeping you stuck, or getting in the way of what you desire. These thoughts run in the background whether you're aware of them or not.

The ten tapping scripts that follow can be used in any order. I suggest you take your time with them to experience the best results. Before tapping, you'll be prompted to think about the topic and rate your level of stress or discomfort on a scale of 1 - 10 (1 = no stress or discomfort, 10 = high stress or discomfort). After each round of tapping, notice how you feel and rate yourself again to see if your number decreased. Continue tapping until you feel some relief. Once your level decreases to a three or below, then move on to the next round of tapping or next script. It may be helpful to have the diagram in front of you until you know the order by heart.

If you're new to Tapping, don't worry. You can't get it wrong. Tapping on each of the tapping points will benefit you and your body. Use the scripts provided to get the feel of Tapping – and don't worry, if some of the phrases don't fit exactly for you, they won't become new problems for you. Like I say when I do Tapping with a group of people, where everyone does Tapping together, "Don't worry, you won't get someone else's problem."

The Tapping topics and scripts that follow have been used successfully for many people. Each script is designed to get to the core of the issue and transform it. Be prepared to make some real, lasting changes, and if there's a thought or a feeling that you can't shift on your own, seek out the assistance of a mental health professional.

1. Stress and Related Symptoms

Think of something you're stressed about and how your body is feeling when you have that thought. Then rate your level of stress on a scale of 1 - 10 (1 = no stress, 10 = high stress). Now you're ready to begin tapping. Tap on each of the tapping points as you say the statements provided or modify the statements to be true for you.

Acknowledging for Stress and Related Symptoms:
EB: This level of stress is not good for me.
SE: I feel the tension in my body.
UE: Sometimes it's difficult to move or breathe.
UN: It's affecting my digestion.
CH: I don't sleep as well as I know I should.
CB: All this stress is taking a toll on my body.
UA: I am under way too much stress.
TH: I am afraid I'm going to end up with a serious illness.
Take a deep breath.

Rate your level of stress again on a scale of 1 - 10. If your level of stress decreased, that's great! If your level of stress increased, that's great too!

Usually, your level of stress will go down, but sometimes it will go up if you got in touch with something that is true for you. All it means is that you have a thought or a feeling telling you something significant.

Of that round of tapping, what stood out the most? Body tension, difficulty moving or breathing, impacted digestion, poor sleep, or fear of ending up with a serious illness? Or did you have a thought about something else?

If your level of stress went up or is between a 7 - 10, I recommend that you do a round of tapping to acknowledge the specific thought or feeling that is keeping it high. Here's an example using the statement, "I'm afraid I'm going to end up with a serious illness."

Acknowledging for a Higher Level of Stress

EB: I feel more stressed.
SE: I'm afraid I'm going to end up with a serious illness.
UE: I don't like this feeling.
UN: I feel stressed at the thought of having a serious illness.
CH: I don't want a serious illness.
CB: If I don't take care of my health, I'm afraid I'm going to end up with a serious illness.
UA: I feel out of control.
TH: Something needs to change.
Take a deep breath.

Rate your level of stress again on a scale of 1 - 10. Did it go down? Did you get clarity about something specific? Your level of stress will continue to go down by tapping and saying statements that you are thinking and feeling. Continue tapping until you feel some relief and your number decreases to a three or below*, before moving on to the possibilities round of tapping.

*You could be ready to move on to the possibility statements if you feel you've done enough acknowledging, even if your level of stress is above a 3. For some people, continuing to talk about something stressful is not helpful, and they do better with possibility statements.

Possibilities for Stress and Related Symptoms:

EB: This level of stress is not sustainable.

SE: I have to do something soon.

UE: Maybe I can learn to relax.

UN: I don't know how that's going to happen.

CH: I know I must do something different.

CB: Maybe I can listen to a guided meditation.

UA: Maybe I can limit my technology time and go to bed at a reasonable time.

TH: Maybe I can do some deep breathing.

Take a deep breath.

Rate your level of stress again on a scale of 1 - 10. Notice any thoughts or feelings that came up or. Continue to tap until you feel some relief before going on to the anchoring statements.

Anchoring for Stress and Related Symptoms:

EB: I am ready to learn how to feel less stressed.

SE: I know I can handle my stress differently.

UE: I can acknowledge how I feel with EFT Tapping.

UN: I can stop and take a deep breath.

CH: I can make a list of things that relax me.

CB: I can do something that brings me joy.

UA: I am ready to manage my stress.

TH: I may even plan a vacation.

Take a deep breath.

Rate your level of stress again on a scale of 1 - 10. By now it should be significantly lower and may even be gone.

2. I Have Too Many Responsibilities

Being responsible is good. Having too many responsibilities isn't. Think about having too many responsibilities and rate your level of stress or discomfort on a scale of 1 - 10.

Acknowledging for I Have Too Many Responsibilities:

EB: Too many people depend on me.

SE: My time and my life are not my own.

UE: It's difficult to even think of putting myself first.

UN: I feel responsible at work and at home.

CH: It's how I was raised.

CB: I don't know how to live any other way.

UA: I am too responsible.

TH: It's not working very well for me.

Take a deep breath.

Rate your level of stress or discomfort again on a scale of 1 - 10 Notice any thoughts or feelings that came up. Continue to tap until you feel some relief before going on to the possibility statements.

Possibilities for I Have Too Many Responsibilities:

EB: Maybe I don't have to do it all.

SE: It's hard to imagine who would do what I do.

UE: I can't keep up this pace.

UN: Something has to change.

CH: There has to be a better way to live.

CB: Maybe I can delegate some responsibilities.

UA: Maybe I can teach others to do what I do.

TH: Maybe I can take some time for myself.

Take a deep breath.

Rate your level of stress or discomfort again on a scale of 1 - 10. Notice any thoughts or feelings that came up. Continue to tap until you feel some relief before going on to the anchoring statements.

Anchoring for I Have Too Many Responsibilities:

EB: I know it's up to me to live my life differently.
SE: If it's going to happen, I have to make it happen.
UE: I am open to figuring out how to live MY life.
UN: Other people seem to live their lives.
CH: It's time to make myself a priority.
CB: Each day I can take 30 minutes for me.
UA: It's a start.
TH: I am ready.
Take a deep breath.

Rate your level of stress or discomfort again on a scale of 1-10. By now it should be significantly lower and may even be gone.

3. I'm Tired

Think about feeling physically or mentally tired or feeling tired of a specific situation that you would like to be different. Rate your level of stress or discomfort on a scale of 1 - 10.

Acknowledging for I'm Tired:

EB: I'm tired.

SE: I'm exhausted.

UE: I'm tired of pretending everything is okay when it's not.

UN: I'm tired of holding it together.

CH: I'm tired of trying to make everyone else happy.

CB: I'm tired of accommodating others.

UA: I'm tired of putting myself and my needs last.

TH: I'm tired.

Take a deep breath.

Rate your level of stress or discomfort again on a scale of 1 - 10. Notice any thoughts or feelings that came up. Continue to tap until you feel some relief before going on to the possibility statements.

Possibilities for I'm Tired:

EB: What would happen if I stopped pretending that I'm okay when I'm not?

SE: What would happen if I thought of myself more often?

UE: Maybe I don't need to worry so much about others.

UN: I wonder what I could do differently?

CH: Maybe I could be honest with myself.

CB: Maybe I could be honest with my family.

UA: Maybe something good will come from this.

TH: I'm ready not to be so tired.

Take a deep breath.

Rate your level of stress or discomfort again on a scale of 1 - 10. Notice any thoughts or feelings that came up. Continue to tap until you feel some relief before going on to the anchoring statements.

Anchoring for I'm Tired:
EB: I know it's up to me to care for my health and happiness.
SE: I am ready to start thinking of MY well-being.
UE: I know I can take better care of me.
UN: I do want to feel healthy and happy.
CH: I give myself permission to do more things for me.
CB: I can speak up more and ask for what I need.
UA: I deserve to be healthy and happy.
TH: I am ready to do more for me.
Take a deep breath.

Rate your level of stress or discomfort again on a scale of 1 - 10. By now it should be significantly lower and may even be gone.

4. Tapping for Sleep

There are two ways you can use this tapping script for sleep. One is to prepare yourself to go to sleep before you've gotten into bed, and the other is while lying in bed unable to fall asleep or unable to go back to sleep.

If you haven't gotten into bed, then use all the tapping points and as much of the script as you feel you need. Once laying down in bed, you may find it too stimulating to use all the tapping points if you are close to falling asleep. In that case, then tap lightly and slowly on the eyebrow, side of the eye, and under the eye points as you say the statements.

Think about having difficulty sleeping and rate your level of stress or discomfort on a scale of 1 - 10.

Acknowledging for Sleep:
EB: I haven't been able to sleep well.
SE: I really need to get some sleep.
UE: I don't believe I can get a good night sleep.
UN: I need to sleep well tonight.
CH: I have too much on my mind.
CB: I want to fall asleep easily.
UA: It's time to go to sleep.
TH: I want to get a good night sleep.
Take a deep breath.

Rate your level of stress or discomfort again on a scale of 1 – 10. Notice any thoughts or feelings that came up. Continue to tap until you feel some relief before going on to the possibility statements.

Remember to say what's true for you as you continue tapping. The tapping will be most effective when you acknowledge your thoughts and feelings.

Possibilities for Sleep:
EB: I wonder how I can get a good night sleep?
SE: I want to believe I can fall asleep easily.
UE: I wonder what it would take to sleep well tonight?
UN: I don't know, but I'm open to something that will work.
CH: Maybe I would sleep better if I believe it's possible to.
CB: Maybe I can let go and surrender to a night of good sleep.
UA: Maybe I could think of something pleasant as I sink into my bed and drift off to sleep.
TH: Maybe I could get a good night sleep tonight.
Take a deep breath.

Rate your level of stress or discomfort again on a scale of 1 - 10. Notice any thoughts or feelings that came up. Continue to tap until you feel some relief before going on to the anchoring statements.

Anchoring for Sleep:
EB: I'm ready for a good night sleep.
SE: There's nothing I have to do at this hour.
UE: Everything I need to do can wait until morning.
UN: There's nowhere else I need to be, except here in bed.
CH: I can surrender to a night of good sleep.
CB: It's my time to sleep and rejuvenate.
UA: I know I will function better with good sleep.
TH: I'm ready for a good night sleep.
Take a deep breath.

Rate your level of stress or discomfort again on a scale of 1 - 10. By now it should be significantly lower and may even be gone.

5. I Don't Want to Feel Deprived

Think about not wanting to feel deprived; not wanting to do without your favorite food, an item, or an activity, then rate your level of stress or discomfort on a scale of 1 - 10. The following tapping scripts use food, but you can substitute it for anything you don't want to feel deprived of.

Acknowledging for I Don't Want to Feel Deprived:
EB: I am not going to give up my favorite food.
SE: What's the joy in that?
UE: I don't want to feel deprived.
UN: I would rather be unhealthy than give up my favorite food.
CH: Food is my friend.
CB: It brings me comfort.
UA: I am not going to give it up.
TH: I don't want to feel deprived.
Take a deep breath.

Rate your level of stress or discomfort again on a scale of 1 - 10. Notice any thoughts or feelings that came up. Continue to tap until you feel some relief before going on to the possibility statements.

Possibilities for I Don't Want to Feel Deprived:
EB: Maybe I don't have to give up my favorite food.
SE: I wonder if I could eat it in moderation.
UE: I want what I want when I want it.
UN: I am not going to deprive myself of the joy of eating.
CH: It is up to me, what, when, and how much I eat.
CB: I get to decide.
UA: Maybe I wouldn't feel deprived if I looked at eating differently.

TH: Maybe I could find comfort and joy in other areas of my life.
Take a deep breath.

Rate your level of stress or discomfort again on a scale of 1 - 10. Notice any thoughts or feelings that came up. Continue to tap until you feel some relief before going on to the anchoring statements.

Anchoring for I Don't Want to Feel Deprived:
EB: It's not all or nothing.
SE: No one is forcing me to give up the foods I enjoy.
UE: I am in control of what I eat.
UN: If I want something, I can have it.
CH: I don't have to feel deprived.
CB: It's okay to want and to have comfort food.
UA: I don't have to have it every day.
TH: I can have what I choose.
Take a deep breath.

Rate your level of stress or discomfort again on a scale of 1 - 10. By now it should be significantly lower and may even be gone.

6. Indulging

Indulging is a behavior most people aren't proud of. Indulging comes from the thought of needing something. It can look and feel like you're out of control – unable to resist, and then leave you feeling bad about yourself. Indulging is a way of coping, and once you know that you are okay, it's possible to let go of this pattern. Be gentle with yourself as you move through these tapping scripts.

Think about indulging with more than you need of something specific just because you want it. Indulging can be with food, alcohol, spending, buying clothes, shoes or makeup, gambling, or anything else in excess, which could result in feeling hardship or distress. Then rate your level of stress or discomfort on a scale of 1 - 10.

Acknowledging for Indulging:
EB: I like to indulge.
SE: Sometimes I can't help it.
UE: Sometimes I can't resist.
UN: I don't feel good after I indulge.
CH: I wish I had more self-control.
CB: I regret indulging.
UA: I feel guilty after indulging.
TH: I wish I had more willpower.
Take a deep breath.

Rate your level of stress or discomfort again on a scale of 1 - 10. Notice any thoughts or feelings that came up. Continue to tap until you feel some relief before going on to the possibility statements.

Possibilities for Indulging:

EB: I wonder if it's possible to have more self-control?

SE: Maybe there is another way of looking at indulging.

UE: What if I didn't worry there wouldn't be enough?

UN: What if I didn't approach indulging from a place of feeling deprived?

CH: I wonder what I can do to have a healthy amount of food or spend a reasonable amount of money without feeling deprived?

CB: Maybe I could be mindful of my eating and spending.

UA: I could remind myself how bad I feel when I indulge.

TH: I could reassure myself that I don't need to indulge.

Take a deep breath.

Rate your level of stress or discomfort again on a scale of 1 - 10. Notice any thoughts or feelings that came up. Continue to tap until you feel some relief before going on to the anchoring statements.

Anchoring for Indulging:

EB: I don't have to be perfect.

SE: I can choose to indulge if I want to.

UE: I am fully aware of how bad I feel when I indulge.

UN: I give myself permission to not indulge.

CH: I trust that I will be able to replace indulging with something healthier.

CB: Indulging is a habit I can overcome with awareness.

UA: Indulging is a habit I can overcome with planning.

TH: I can make a list of things I could do when I want to indulge.

Take a deep breath.

Rate your level of stress or discomfort again on a scale of 1 - 10. By now it should be significantly lower and may even be gone.

7. I Want What I Want When I Want It

Have you ever had the thought, "I want it now, and nobody is going to tell me I can't have it." Several clients I've worked with have used the expression, "I want what I want when I want it." There are many reasons why someone would feel so strongly about wanting something. The tapping scripts that follow will guide you through common thoughts you may be having about wanting what you want when you want it, and possible solutions. Be patient with yourself as you do the tapping. This pattern of thinking has probably been with you for a very long time.

Think about wanting what you want when you want it and rate your level of stress or discomfort on a scale of 1 - 10.

Acknowledging for I Want What I Want When I Want It:
EB: I want it.
SE: No one is going to tell me I can't have it.
UE: I want it.
UN: I want to eat things that aren't good for me.
CH: I want to buy things I can't afford.
CB: I will fight for what I know I shouldn't have.
UA: When I am told I can't, I get defensive and want it more.
TH: I want it.
Take a deep breath.

Rate your level of stress or discomfort again on a scale of 1 – 10. Notice any thoughts or feelings that came up. Continue to tap until you feel some relief before going on to the possibility statements.

Possibilities for I Want What I Want When I Want It:

EB: Could it be that I am rebellious?

SE: Maybe this is a way of having some control over my life.

UE: There must be a reason why I want what I want.

UN: I think this is safer than expressing my feelings.

CH: I am afraid of my feelings.

CB: Maybe I could be honest with myself and how I feel.

UA: Maybe I could write down my thoughts and feelings.

TH: Maybe I could find another outlet for my feelings.

Take a deep breath.

Rate your level of stress or discomfort again on a scale of 1 - 10. Notice any thoughts or feelings that came up. Continue to tap until you feel some relief before going on to the anchoring statements.

Anchoring for I Want What I Want When I Want It:

EB: I am free to choose.

SE: I can want something and think about it before acting.

UE: I don't have to defend my choices.

UN: I can choose to eat or buy whatever I want.

CH: I can deal with my feelings differently

CB: It's my choice.

UA: I don't have to be rebellious to get my needs met.

TH: I can make my own decisions that are right for me.

Take a deep breath.

Rate your level of stress or discomfort again on a scale of 1 - 10. By now it should be significantly lower and may even be gone.

8. I Feel Ashamed of My Body

There's a reason why people let themselves go and treat themselves poorly. It's not because of a poor diet and lack of exercise. There's always something deeper going on.

Shame is a feeling that you are bad in some way, and when you feel shame, it's easy to give up on yourself. You may not have gotten the validation you needed growing up to feel good about yourself and your body. It's never too late to change the way you think and feel about your body.

Be honest with yourself and the way you feel about your body. Think about feeling ashamed of your body, a part of your body, or the health of your body, then rate your level of stress or discomfort on a scale of 1 - 10.

Acknowledging for I Feel Ashamed of My Body:
EB: I can't believe this is me.
SE: I let myself go.
UE: I feel ashamed of the way I look.
UN: I have no self-control.
CH: I never intended to look like this.
CB: It happened.
UA: I feel so ashamed.
TH: I don't like feeling this way.
Take a deep breath.

Rate your level of stress or discomfort again on a scale of 1 – 10. Notice any thoughts or feelings that came up. Continue to tap until you feel some relief before going on to the possibility statements.

Possibilities for I Feel Ashamed of My Body:

EB: I wonder if it's possible to ever like my body.

SE: I have a hard time accepting the way I look.

UE: I wonder if I could ever like my body.

UN: I wonder what it would take to like myself.

CH: There has to be a way to look and feel better.

CB: Maybe I could find one thing to like about my body.

UA: Maybe I could be more kind to myself and my body.

TH: Maybe I could do something nice for myself.

Take a deep breath.

Rate your level of stress or discomfort again on a scale of 1 - 10. Notice any thoughts or feelings that came up. Continue to tap until you feel some relief before going on to the anchoring statements.

Anchoring for I Feel Ashamed of My Body:

EB: I wouldn't treat a friend the way I treat myself.

SE: There are lots of things I could do for myself.

UE: I am ready to be my own best friend.

UN: I am willing to stop the negative comments about myself.

CH: I am ready to treat myself with respect.

CB: It is up to me to begin to like myself and my body.

UA: It's time for me to take charge of my body.

TH: It is up to me to begin to like myself and my body.

Take a deep breath.

Rate your level of stress or discomfort again on a scale of 1 - 10. By now it should be significantly lower and may even be gone.

9. I Can't Stick with a Plan

There's always something bigger at play when you want something and can't make it happen. If you don't believe it's possible to stick with a plan, because of your past experiences, that belief will interfere with your efforts.

The tapping scripts for this topic are to move you from feeling like you can't stick with something, to feeling like it's possible. You may have some resistance come up. Resistance expected when you have an inner conflict between what you want and your subconscious protecting you from another negative experience.

Think about not being able to stick with a plan and rate your level of stress or discomfort on a scale of 1 - 10.

Acknowledging for I Can't Stick with a Plan:
EB: I have tried everything.
SE: I failed.
UE: I feel like giving up.
UN: I haven't been able to stick with a plan.
CH: I don't know why it has to be so hard.
CB: I have a pattern of being inconsistent.
UA: It's no use.
TH: Nothing ever works for me.
Take a deep breath.

Rate your level of stress or discomfort again on a scale of 1 - 10. Notice any thoughts or feelings that came up. Continue to tap until you feel some relief before going on to the possibility statements.

Possibilities for I Can't Stick with a Plan:

EB: I want to do better and maybe I can.

SE: I want to be healthier.

UE: What if I could become healthier?

UN: Maybe I can acknowledge what's getting in the way.

CH: What if I could let go of the thoughts I have, that I can't?

CB: Maybe I could start small.

UA: Maybe I could try one new thing.

TH: Maybe I could believe in myself.

Take a deep breath.

Rate your level of stress or discomfort again on a scale of 1 - 10. Notice any thoughts or feelings that came up. Continue to tap until you feel some relief before going on to the anchoring statements.

Anchoring for I Can't Stick with a Plan:

EB: I am ready to live a life less burdened by my past.

SE: I am ready to live like the slim, healthy person I am becoming.

UE: I am ready to treat my body and myself with loving care.

UN: I don't have to do it all at once.

CH: I can go at my pace.

CB: I can make one small change today.

UA: I can be realistic and steadily do what it takes.

TH: I know what to do and I know I can do it.

Take a deep breath.

Rate your level of stress or discomfort again on a scale of 1 - 10. By now it should be significantly lower and may even be gone.

10. I'm Afraid to Lose Weight

It's not uncommon to be afraid to lose weight. I've worked with many clients who say they feel safer in a bigger body. Added weight can be a protective barrier for anyone who has been abused or wants to avoid intimacy. If you can relate, and it feels like too big of an issue to deal with on your own, I highly suggest you seek out help.

For people who have successfully lost weight and gained it back, or who desire to lose weight, but question if they can sustain a weight loss, the fear is real. For others, the fear of being seen or attracting attention is a factor.

Think about being afraid to lose weight and rate your level of stress or discomfort on a scale of 1 - 10.

Acknowledging for I'm Afraid to Lose Weight:
EB: The thought of losing weight is scary.
SE: It's too much pressure.
UE: Then I have to maintain it.
UN: What if I gain it all back?
CH: I am not ready to lose weight and attract attention to myself.
CB: Losing weight will change my relationship with people.
UA: It's too scary.
TH: I am afraid to lose weight.
Take a deep breath.

Rate your level of stress or discomfort again on a scale of 1 – 10. Notice any thoughts or feelings that came up. Continue to tap until you feel some relief before going on to the possibility statements.

Possibilities for I'm Afraid to Lose Weight:

EB: I wonder what would happen if I wasn't so afraid of losing weight.

SE: I wonder if I'm ready?

UE: I may need to look at my fears and face them.

UN: It's possible that if I lost weight, I wouldn't feel these fears.

CH: Maybe it doesn't have to be so scary.

CB: Maybe I can lose weight with ease.

UA: Maybe I can get support along the way.

TH: Maybe it will feel good to be seen.

Take a deep breath.

Rate your level of stress or discomfort again on a scale of 1 - 10. Notice any thoughts or feelings that came up. Continue to tap until you feel some relief before going on to the anchoring statements.

Anchoring for I'm Afraid to Lose Weight:

EB: I am ready to become healthier by losing weight.

SE: I am willing to take the risk of losing weight.

UE: I can get support and help with the process.

UN: I know I am not alone in this.

CH: I don't need to worry about things that I imagine.

CB: I'm ready to make a change and do it for me.

UA: It's time for me to lose weight.

TH: I don't need the extra baggage anymore.

Take a deep breath.

Rate your level of stress or discomfort again on a scale of 1 - 10. By now it should be significantly lower and may even be gone.

Take Action:

EFT Tapping is highly effective in calming the flight or fight response, reducing stress, and releasing stored emotions.

Below are some suggestions to make EFT Tapping more effective, and how to use tapping for other situations:

1. For additional support with EFT Tapping visit my website at https://www.phyllisginsberg.com/tapping-with-phyllis.

2. The more specific your statements are to you, the more effective the tapping will be. Feel free to modify any of the phrases to express your thoughts and feelings more accurately.

3. Always start by acknowledging your thoughts and feelings. You can do additional tapping on any thought or feeling you have. Simply say what you are thinking or feeling as you do the tapping.

4. Make a list of the messages you heard as a child from the people who raised you. They could be about you, your body, or food. For each statement, list a few thoughts and feelings you have about it. Then choose one statement group and tap on each of the tapping points as you say the statement and your thoughts and feelings about it.

5. Seek professional psychological help if needed, to address any thoughts or feelings that you are unable to reduce the severity of on your own.

Part Three: Healthy Sleep

CHAPTER 6

Poor Sleep - What You Need to Know

Sleep is the time when your body repairs itself at the cellular level. What happens when you deprive yourself of this repair time due to sleepless nights? Lack of sleep has been linked to increased rates of heart disease, obesity, stroke, and even certain types of cancers. If that isn't enough, multiple nights of poor sleep can affect your mental performance, ability to learn, and to problem solve.[1]

The most vital repair of your body happens when you are in a deep sleep, mainly during the first half of the night. Deep slow-wave sleep is the stage that is the deepest, most restful, and most restorative. Growth hormones are released during sleep. This is when children grow taller, your skin cells regenerate, and your hair gets longer.

While you sleep, the hormones that regulate appetite are released, and muscles are repaired from damage and wear and tear from the day.

Sleep also plays an integral role in regulating the body's immune system, which is responsible for fighting off everything from the common cold to more serious chronic problems like cancer. Studies show that individuals are more likely to catch a cold virus when sleep deprived. Research suggests that the body produces fewer infection-fighting antibodies when sleep deprived.[2]

3 Key Reasons Your Brain Needs Sleep

As we rest our head upon cushy pillows at night, we don't typically think about our brain. But as we drop off to sleep, our brain begins to get to work, on behalf of the emotions and physical health that are important to our very survival! Here is just some of what your brain is doing for you while you're in dreamland:

1. "Quality REM (Rapid Eye Movement) sleep lets your brain consolidate memories and improves cognition," says Raj Dasgupta, M.D., professor and sleep physician at the Keck School of Medicine of USC. Dreaming in REM also appears to be when the brain puts emotional events into perspective – not just recently encountered information, but also selectively preserving in memory what is most important and beneficial to us.[3]

2. Sleep helps your brain keep your attention and focus sharp. You know that "foggy" feeling when you haven't had enough sleep, and you just can't pay attention like you usually do? Your brain needs more sleep!

3. Your brain, which regulates mood and coping skills, needs a good night's sleep to work optimally. Chronic insomnia has been linked to increased risk of developing a mood disorder, such as anxiety or depression.[4]

Sleep and Your Fat Cells

Sleep has been shown to affect your fat cells! A study from the University of Chicago, published in the *Annals of Internal Medicine*, determined that four nights of sleep deprivation reduced insulin sensitivity in fat cells by a whopping 30%.[5]

The less sensitive your cells are to insulin, the less your body produces the hunger-regulating hormone leptin. The less leptin you produce, the hungrier you are, and the sensors that tell you when you are full or satisfied don't work properly. At the same time, your body may produce higher levels of ghrelin, a biochemical that stimulates appetite. As a result, you may experience food cravings even after you've eaten an adequate number of calories, leading to overeating and weight gain or difficulty losing weight.[6]

It only takes two or three nights of poor sleep to feel sleep deprived. Sleep deprivation is a serious problem that affects every area of life, from your food choices to your ability to be productive, attentive, and healthy.

Difficulty falling asleep and difficulty staying asleep are common problems for millions of people. More than a third of American adults are not getting enough sleep on a regular basis, according to a study in the Centers for Disease Control and Prevention's (CDC) Morbidity and Mortality Weekly Report.[7]

The American Academy of Sleep Medicine and the Sleep Research Society recommend that adults aged 18–60 sleep at least 7 hours each night to promote optimal health and well-being. Sleeping less than seven hours per day is associated with an increased risk of developing chronic conditions such as obesity, diabetes, high blood pressure, heart disease, stroke, and frequent mental distress.[8]

Sleep Challenges

If you want to sleep better, stop working! Well, that may not be possible, of course, but in all seriousness, the main reason many of us are sleeping so little is that Americans are working longer – an average of 44 hours per week. And a record 17% of U.S. adults now log 60 or more hours per week in the office, leaving less time for sleep.

Working longer hours, plus having longer commutes, leaves less time for domestic chores, like paying bills, which get pushed into evening time. In today's global economy, working late into the night or first thing in the morning is often a necessity. That kind of shift work, which was once mainly confined to nurses, emergency room doctors, factory workers, and police officers, can wreak havoc on the body's sleep-wake cycle.

And then there are modern habits like staying up late using electronic devices, even as research suggests that blue light from those devices may interfere with the body's production of melatonin, the sleep hormone.[9]

What can you do without quitting your job? Make sleep a priority!

Take Action:

The benefits of sleep are undeniable. Sleep is vital for your mental, emotional, and physical health.

Do one or more of the following to get adequate sleep:

1. Calculate when you would need to fall asleep to get the recommended seven hours of sleep each night. Then aim to go to bed at least 30 minutes before the time you want to be asleep.

2. If you tend to be a night owl and you have trouble falling asleep earlier, try going to bed 30 minutes earlier than your regular bedtime for a few nights, then 30 minutes earlier from that time. Do this until you are sleeping the recommended seven hours a night.

3. Try Tapping for Sleep (on page 57) to calm your thoughts and your body so that you can fall asleep more easily.

Notes

[1] The Link Between Sleep Duration and Chronic Disease.
http://healthysleep.med.harvard.edu/healthy/matters/consequences/sleep-and-disease-risk

[2] What Happens in Your Body and Brain While You Sleep
https://www.nbcnews.com/better/health/what-happens-your-body-brain-while-you-sleep-ncna805276

[3] REM Sleep Enhances Emotional Memories, Study Shows
https://news.nd.edu/news/rem-sleep-enhances-emotional-memories-study-shows/

[4] Sleep Deprivation Can Cause Anxiety and Depression and the Problem Goes Both Ways
https://qz.com/986110/sleep-deprivation-can-cause-anxiety-and-depression-and-the-problem-goes-both-ways

[5] Even Your Fat Cells Need Sleep
https://news.uchicago.edu/story/even-your-fat-cells-need-sleep-according-new-research

[6] Why Sleep Is the Number 1 Most Important Thing to a Better Body
https://www.shape.com/lifestyle/mind-and-body/why-sleep-no-1-most-important-thing-better-body

[7] Short Sleep Duration Among US Adults
https://www.cdc.gov/sleep/data_statistics.html

---

[8] One In Three Adults Don't Get Enough Sleep
https://www.cdc.gov/media/releases/2016/p0215-enough-sleep.html

[9] Why Americans Can't Sleep
https://www.consumerreports.org/sleep/why-americans-cant-sleep

CHAPTER 7

Melatonin, the Sleep Hormone

Melatonin is a hormone that regulates your sleep, wakefulness, and circadian rhythm. Circadian rhythm describes the sleep/wake cycle, a biological clock that runs in your brain and cycles between sleepiness and alertness. It explains why you may feel energized or sleepy at around the same time each day. Secretion of melatonin is low during daylight, ascending after the onset of darkness, peaking in the middle of the night between 11 PM and 3 AM, and then falling sharply before the time of light onset.

Studies have shown that melatonin supplementation may positively affect several measures of sleep. A systematic analysis of several placebo-controlled studies showed that melatonin treatment significantly reduced sleep onset latency, increased sleep efficiency, and increased total sleep duration. It's recommended to take melatonin 30 - 60 minutes before sleep. If you are a night owl and usually go to bed late, you may want to take melatonin 2 - 3 hours before your desired bedtime, if you want to go to sleep earlier than usual.[1]

The research on how much melatonin to take ranges from 0.1mg – 10mg. A high dose of melatonin could cause side effects including a headache, short-term feelings of depression, daytime sleepiness, dizziness, stomach cramps, and irritability.[2] Check with your health care provider to see if a melatonin supplement is advised, and the recommended dosage for you.

How to Increase Melatonin Naturally

Before you go out and buy melatonin, you might try doing a couple of things that could naturally increase the production of your melatonin.

Exposure to light, especially blue light from electronics (cell phone, television, computer, tablet, and fluorescent lights), may cause you to have difficulty falling asleep and staying asleep. These lights have your brain thinking that it's daytime and not the time to produce melatonin for sleep. Avoid using electronic devices at night before going to sleep. Experiment with decreasing your exposure to unnecessary light 30 - 90 minutes before you want to go to sleep.

If you can't bear the thought of not watching your favorite television shows at night or being on your smartphone, tablet, or computer, there are blue-light-blocking glasses that can be worn to prevent the disruption of sleep due to blue light from screens. Cathy Goldstein, an assistant professor of neurology at the University of Michigan Sleep Disorders Center, says that when blue-light-blocking glasses are used, the light doesn't suppress your melatonin and it can improve sleep.

There's a growing body of research to back up the claim that blocking blue light before bed can help you sleep better. In one study, from 2009, volunteers who wore blue-light-blocking glasses three hours before bedtime reported better sleep quality and mood than those who didn't. A more recent study of teenage boys found similar results.[3]

Caffeine Suppresses Melatonin

You may not have to give up your coffee, tea, soda, or chocolate, but consider this if you have a difficult time falling asleep; it could be due to your caffeine consumption. Caffeine can disrupt your normal sleep-wake cycle. It might surprise you to hear, but caffeine has an even stronger influence on melatonin suppression than bright light.

The effects of caffeine can last in your body for several hours. It can take from 6 - 8 hours for the stimulant effects of caffeine to be reduced by one half. When it comes to daily caffeine intake, it's important to think about the amount of caffeine and the time of day you're consuming it. Also consider that you might be consuming multiple sources of caffeine, increasing your total amount for the day.[4]

Morning Sunlight and Sleep

Sunlight and darkness signal the release of hormones in your brain. Exposure to sunlight increases the release of serotonin, the hormone associated with elevating mood and helping you feel calm and focused. At night, as it gets darker, the brain produces the sleep hormone, melatonin. Ideally, the production of serotonin and melatonin occur to have you awake and alert in the morning and sleepy at night.

Unfortunately, without enough sun exposure, serotonin levels can decline, making it difficult to wake up in the morning. People with very low levels of serotonin may experience seasonal affect disorder (SAD) and feel depressed during dark winter months.[5]

You don't have to have SAD to benefit from morning sunlight or Light Therapy. When your body is in sync with nature's light-dark cycle, your production of melatonin will regulate, making it easier to fall asleep at night.

It is recommended to expose your eyes to light upon waking or shortly after. Open the shades and let the sunlight in or better yet, go outside for natural sunlight. Do not look directly at the sun. If where you live there isn't enough natural sunlight or if you suffer from SAD, then Light Therapy is usually administered in the morning based on the regular waking time. Those with seasonal depression are typically given a dose of 10,000 lux for 30 minutes shortly after awakening. Morning light therapy seems to work by advancing the circadian rhythm. That is, it helps people feel sleepy earlier and get up earlier. This seems to occur because the light exposure shifts the time at which melatonin is released in the evening.[6]

Take Action:

Melatonin is essential for quality sleep. It's what regulates your sleep/wake cycle. There are several ways to increase your melatonin naturally, or you could take a melatonin supplement.

Try one or more of the following to increase your melatonin levels:

1. Get sun or light exposure first thing in the morning with natural light or a lightbox.

2. Avoid using electronics with blue light 30 - 90 minutes before you want to go to sleep.

3. Wear blue-light-blocker glasses if you are using electronics in the evening.

4. Be mindful of your caffeine intake from all sources and eliminate the consumption of caffeine 6 - 8 hours before bedtime.

5. Ask your health care provider about taking a melatonin supplement and the dosage recommended for you.

Notes

[1] 15 Questions About Melatonin and Sleep
https://www.docsopinion.com/2018/04/02/melatonin-sleep-melatonin-supplements/

[2] Melatonin Side Effects
https://www.webmd.com/vitamins/ai/ingredientmono-940/melatonin

[3] Melatonin Side Effects
https://www.webmd.com/vitamins/ai/ingredientmono-940/melatonin

[4] Is Caffeine Causing Your Sleeplessness?
https://www.thesleepdoctor.com/2017/08/31/caffeine-causing-sleeplessness

[5] What Are the Benefits of Sunlight?
https://www.healthline.com/health/depression/benefits-sunlight

[6] Light Therapy
https://www.psychologytoday.com/us/blog/sleepless-in-america/201101/light-therapy

CHAPTER 8

How to Consistently Get Good Sleep

Keep it cool to get the best night's sleep. Research shows that sleep happens best in a dark, cool room at about 65 degrees. Your body is designed to begin cooling down for sleep, and that begins in late afternoon and continues until the evening hours. Thermoregulation is the process your body goes through on a 24-hour circadian cycle, as does the sleep-wake cycle. The adjustment of your core temperature takes place, lowering your body temperature at night, helping you fall asleep and stay asleep through the night. Rising temperature signals your body to move into a state of alertness in the morning.[1]

Set your thermostat to a comfortable, cool temperature, open a window, or turn on a fan. If you feel cold, wear socks to bed rather than heavy pajamas or piling on blankets. The idea is to be comfortable enough to fall asleep and not get too hot during the night. If you feel too warm when you go to sleep or tend to wake up feeling hot, wear light, breathable nightwear.

What About a Relaxing Bath?

A hot bath can be just what you need to relax and unwind from the day. Like exercise, hot baths and showers can help you fall asleep. The problem, however, comes when taking one too close to the time you plan on going to sleep. Being overheated or sweating can make it difficult to sleep. Let your body cool down before heading off to bed. Some people need 60 - 90 minutes to cool down.[2]

Three Steps to a Better Night's Sleep

Worrying and feeling tense or stressed at bedtime can make it difficult to fall asleep, but having trouble falling asleep, and in turn, not getting enough sleep, can also result in feeling anxious. Anxiety can lead to sleep problems, insomnia in particular, and sleep problems can lead to anxiety.[3] Not a healthy cycle to be in!

Here are three steps to help you get a better night's sleep:

Step 1: To put your thoughts and worries to rest, take a few minutes before bed and write them down. Include any concerns you have about sleep as well. Then write a "to do" list for the next day. All those things will be waiting for you when you wake up, so no need to visit them during the night.

Step 2: Next, just before turning off the light, write 3 - 5 of your happiest moments of the day in a journal or notebook. Your happiest moments will shift your brain to thinking about pleasant things before drifting off to sleep.

Step 3: Turn out the light and surrender to a night of restful sleep. Know that there is nowhere you need to go and nothing you need to do. Night time is your time to sleep and allow your body to rest and rejuvenate.

Sweet dreams tonight!

Do's and Don'ts for Better Sleep

- ❖ Ideally, it's best to begin winding down your activities and your mind an hour or two before going to bed.

- ❖ Find ways to relax in the evening with quiet activities; read a book or magazine, do a puzzle, have calm conversations, do some yoga or stretching. Listen to calm music, meditate, or do slow deep breathing.

- ❖ Keep your sleeping space neat, clean, and at a cool temperature.

- ❖ Create a bedtime routine that lets your body know it is time to unwind and get ready for sleep. Choose the order of what you do before bed. Wash your face, brush your teeth, change into nightclothes...

- ❖ Get up at the same hour each morning. By training your body to get up at a set time each day, even on weekends, you will naturally fall into a regular bedtime that corresponds to your body's need for sleep. Some days you'll need more sleep at night. Listen to your body, go to bed early if you are tired and avoid staying up too late. When you feel sleepy, it's your body's way of telling you it needs rest.

- Stressful conversations before bed can leave you agitated, making it difficult to fall asleep or stay asleep. Avoid participating in or watching others engage in conflict, including what you watch on television, in a movie, or on the news.

- Refrain from doing things that will stimulate your mind or keep you awake close to bedtime. Before bed is not the time to be reading a book that you can't put down.

- It's best to avoid exposure to blue light from electronics an hour or two before bed. If you must use electronics, blue-light-blocking glasses could help.

- Use the EFT Tapping script for sleep (on page 57).

- Going to bed on a full stomach can cause insomnia and heartburn. It's advised to wait 2 - 3 hours for food to digest before lying down and going to sleep.[4]

- Consuming large amounts of liquids an hour or two before bed will increase the need to use the toilet in the middle of the night. Drink liquids earlier in the evening to give yourself time to empty your bladder before going to bed.

- The consumption of caffeine, tobacco, alcohol, and other stimulants may disrupt your sleep. Depending on your sensitivity, these can have a negative impact on your sleep. It's wise to limit your caffeine consumption to a small amount early in the day if you have trouble sleeping.

Take Action:

To get a restful night of sleep, it's important to be calm, comfortable, and sleepy when you are ready to go to bed.

Try one or more of the numerous suggestions from this chapter to help you sleep better:

1. Put your thoughts and worries to rest by using the Three Steps to a Better Night's Sleep (on page 88).

2. Review the Do's and Don'ts for Better Sleep (on page 89). Select one or two remedies that you can easily do. Experiment with some of the others, if necessary, until you're sleeping well.

Notes

[1] Optimal Sleep Temperature and The Role of Thermoregulation in Sleeping Through the Night
https://www.thesleepdoctor.com/2018/04/01/chilipad/

[2] Eight Things You Shouldn't Do Before Bed
https://www.care2.com/greenliving/stop-doing-these-things-before-sleep.html

[3] Sleep Deprivation Can Cause Anxiety and Depression, and the Problem Goes Both Ways.
http://theconversation.com/theres-a-strong-link-between-anxiety-and-depression-and-sleep-problems-and-it-goes-both-ways-76145

[4] Eating Before Bed
https://www.verywellhealth.com/eating-before-bed-3014981

Part Four: Healthy Body

CHAPTER 9

How to Work with Your Body

The best way to start getting healthier is to listen to your body – your body KNOWS how to heal and how to thrive. And when it does, you do too!

How carefully do you listen to your body? Do you notice the first signs of stress, discomfort, minor aches or pains, or a change in mood? If so, do you brush it off and press on? Our culture has been more focused on "doing" rather than "being," and "results before feelings."

Sometimes it takes a major crisis to get us to slow down or stop and really look at how we are living our lives. You have a miraculous body that can give you guidance and messages if you take the time to listen. Try using the following Four Steps to Tuning in to Your Body's Signals when something doesn't feel right, or as a daily practice.

Four Steps to Tuning in to Your Body's Signals

1. Stop for a moment.

2. Tune in to how you feel.

3. Scan your body for discomfort.

4. Ask yourself what you need.

It can be this simple. Often, by acknowledging how you feel, and by asking what you need, you can reduce symptoms and gain insight into a better way of doing, being, or living.

Is Your Body a Pond or a River?

Have you ever seen a body of water, like a pond that has no water flowing into it or going out from it? It just stands there with no movement. It looks dirty and may have algae, dirt, and leaves in it. In contrast, a river is a naturally flowing source of fresh water, heading toward a lake or ocean.

Movement of your body is like the water of a flowing river. When you have good circulation from movement, your body can function optimally. Lack of movement, like a stagnant pond with no motion, can put a strain on your circulatory systems and leave you feeling sluggish.

Physical activity gets your heart pumping blood throughout your body, carrying oxygen and nutrients to where they are needed. Take just 15 - 30 minutes, once or twice a day, and do of any form of exercise or movement you enjoy. It will improve your digestion, mood, energy, sleep, and allow you to maintain a healthy body weight or lose weight.[1] Movement, along with proper nutrition and plenty of water, will keep your body functioning at its best.

Stand Up – It's Good For You!

Research has linked sitting for long periods of time with several health concerns, such as obesity, increased blood pressure, high blood sugar, excess body fat around the waist, and abnormal cholesterol levels. Too much sitting overall and prolonged periods of sitting also seem to increase the risk of death from cardiovascular disease and cancer. [2]

Sitting for long periods, especially at the computer, can cause your body to become stiff, sore, and lethargic. Have you noticed your posture when you sit for hours? Your body was designed to move, not sit at a desk.

When you sit, you use less energy than you do when you stand or move. Any extended sitting, such as at a desk, behind the wheel of a car, or in front of a TV screen or monitor, can be harmful. An analysis of 13 studies of sitting time and activity levels found that those who sat for more than eight hours a day with no physical activity had a risk of death similar to the risks of dying posed by obesity and smoking. However, unlike some other studies, this analysis of data from more than 1 million people found that 60 to 75 minutes of moderately intense physical activity a day countered the effects of too much sitting. Another study found that sitting time contributed little to mortality for people who were most active.[3]

At the very least, take a stretch break every 30 - 60 minutes, walk around, gently reach for the sky, do shoulder shrugs, march in place, walk a flight of stairs, or go outside for a 5 - 10-minute walk. Preventative medicine doctor Robert Corish, M.D., says, "The more you can get up and move, the better. Even short breaks of standing up, stretching and walking during the work day will make a significant difference in your health outcome and disease reduction."

Recovering from Back Pain

An estimated 80% of adults will experience back pain at some point. Most of us don't learn how to take care of our backs until we have a back injury. When I was in my late 20s, I was pushing a shopping cart full of groceries with my 4-year-old daughter in it. We were in a new area, and I didn't see the potholes in the parking lot. The shopping cart started to tip, and I used all my strength to keep the cart upright. The next thing I knew, I had a severe back injury. I was in pain for almost two years with a soft tissue injury. Chiropractic treatment gave me temporary relief. I was finally referred to an orthopedic surgeon who gave me a booklet of back exercises, which I did daily, and within a short time, I was pain-free. My theory is that I continued to have back pain because I was not told to strengthen my core, which ultimately gave me the support I needed to heal from the original back injury.

Here are some tips to help you prevent and recover from back pain:

1. First, get an assessment of your back pain or injury, so you know your condition. Then, if given the okay from your doctor, try specific back exercises. Ask your doctor, chiropractor, personal trainer, or physical therapist, for back and core strengthening exercises.

2. Get regular movement. People who exercise regularly tend to have less back pain. Do low-impact activities, like walking or swimming, restorative yoga or take a Feldenkrais (Awareness Through Movement) class. These will get more blood flowing to your back muscles for repair and healing.

3. When lifting, bend with your knees, and spread your legs in a wide stance for more stability. Hold objects close to your body; it puts less strain on your back. And when in doubt, ask for help.

4. Take a stretch break every 30 - 60 minutes from sitting too long at the computer, in the car, or on the couch.

5. Aim to reach and maintain a healthy body weight. Less weight puts less of a strain on your back.

Stress, Emotions, and Physical Symptoms

Did you know that the American Medical Association states, **"80% of all health problems are stress related,"** and the Centers for Disease Control and Prevention has stated, **"85% of all diseases appear to have an emotional component?"** This is important information because it impacts everyone! Too much stress and heavy emotions cause physical pain and physical symptoms.

In addition to daily stress, adverse childhood experiences can set us up for health problems throughout our lives, whether or not we are consciously thinking of the experiences.[4] And of course, unresolved feelings of grief, anger, resentment, and fear from childhood experiences may contribute to physical and emotional difficulties.

In Part 1: Healthy Mind, I covered how your thoughts create healthy "feel good" hormones" or unhealthy "stress" hormones. These hormones regulate how your body functions and what genes get turned on and off. If you are suffering from pain or an illness, you may want to go back and re-read Part 1: Healthy Mind (on page 1).

In Part Two: Healthy Energy, I introduced EFT Tapping, a technique that releases stored emotions. When stored emotions are released with tapping, it's not uncommon for physical pain to decrease or go away. The tapping script, "Stress and Related Symptoms," (on page 50), will help you begin to release stuck energy that may be causing pain, discomfort or symptoms.

Lose 7.5 Pounds by Simply Walking

One part of creating a healthy lifestyle is taking care of your body. Did you know that there are benefits to just walking? And it doesn't have to be a fast walk. If you walk for 20 minutes a day, five days a week, you will gain healthful benefits that may include better circulation, more mobility, and better posture. You may even reduce the chance of premature death by between 16% and 30%.[5]

If all you did were 20 minutes of walking five days a week and didn't change your eating habits, you would lose approximately 7.5 pounds in a year. Walking for 20 minutes at a moderate pace burns about

100 calories. That's 500 calories a week, and it takes 3,500 calories to equal one pound.

Get a walking buddy, a friend, your dog, or someone else's dog, or go by yourself, you get the idea. It's only 10 minutes out and 10 minutes back. Start walking!

Take Action:

It's easier to take care of your body when you know how. Listen to your body. It will give you the clues to what it needs to function optimally. Then take action.

Do one or more of the following to work with your body:

1. Notice when you discount a thought, feeling, or symptom in your body.

2. Use the Four Steps to Tuning into Your Body (on page 94). Listen to your body by scanning for any discomfort or mild aches and pains and address them before they become worse.

3. Improve the circulation within your body with movement of any kind. Walk, stretch, take the stairs, do yoga, ride a bike, or another type of movement you enjoy.

4. Avoid sitting too long by setting a timer to go off every 30 - 60 minutes to remind yourself to get up and stretch or walk around.

5. Take a restorative yoga class or Feldenkrais class.

6. To better understand the connection between your thoughts and your body, go back and re-read Part 1: Healthy Mind (on page 1).

7. Use the EFT Tapping script from Chapter 3, "Stress and Related Symptoms," (on page 50). It may be the answer to reducing or eliminating physical pain or symptoms caused by conscious or unconscious emotions.

Notes

[1] How Physical Exercise Makes Your Brain Work Better
https://www.theguardian.com/education/2016/jun/18/how-physical-exercise-makes-your-brain-work-better

Exercise Affects Digestion
https://www.manhattangastroenterology.cowm/exercise-affects-digestion/

[2] What Are the Risks of Sitting Too Much?
https://www.mayoclinic.org/healthy-lifestyle/adult-health/expert-answers/sitting/faq-20058005

[3] What Are the Risks of Sitting Too Much?
https://www.mayoclinic.org/healthy-lifestyle/adult-health/expert-answers/sitting/faq-20058005

[4] Adverse Childhood Experiences
https://www.cdc.gov/violenceprevention/childabuseandneglect/acestudy/index.html

[5] Walking Benefits
http://www.huffingtonpost.ca/2015/01/16/walking-benefits_n_6486906.html

Why Walking Is the Most Underrated Form of Exercise
https://www.nbcnews.com/better/health/why-walking-most-underrated-form-exercise-ncna797271

Walking for Better Back Health
https://www.spine-health.com/wellness/exercise/exercise-walking-better-back-health

CHAPTER 10

Why Go Out of My Way to Exercise?

I have a confession to make. Getting regular exercise has been my biggest downfall. I attribute this to two factors. One was feeling isolated as a child, and the other was that I had no role models. I never saw either of my parents participate in any physical activity. For decades I have struggled with making time for exercise. I didn't, and sometimes still don't, value it enough over all the other things I must do.

I feel great by eating well and have been able to maintain a healthy body weight, so I often don't make exercise a priority. I get plenty of movement, but I don't workout as often as I'd like. The benefits of exercising are so clear and compelling that it's a key part of this book.

Why Exercise?

How about exercising to have a healthy body with good posture, to decrease stress, elevate mood, increase energy, and contribute to a strong, healthy immune system and well-functioning body? Or, to improve strength, flexibility, coordination, and circulation? How about helping with weight loss and weight management?[1] Keep in mind that you can never exercise enough to burn excess calories consumed by indulgent eating or overeating.

The Centers for Disease Control and Prevention recommends that children and adolescents get 60 minutes of physical activity on most, and preferably all, days of the week, and adults should get 2 hours and 30 minutes (150 minutes) of moderate-intensity aerobic activity (brisk walking) every week.[2]

Brain Research and Exercise

Did you know that exercise is highly correlated with the production of new brain cells resulting in improved learning and memory? Brain research has also revealed a correlation between exercise and a decrease in depression.[3] My favorite is that neuroscience has validated children learn better when they engage in daily physical activity.[4] I hope everyone who has children reads this and role models and encourages regular exercise for their children, so they don't struggle with it as I do.

Let's Get Moving

Treat your body to some movement. Find what works for you: walk, run, swim, jog, bike, skate, ski, use a treadmill, rowing machine, elliptical, stair climber, mini-trampoline, video, or attend classes, do yoga... Or, put on some music and dance. Just get moving!

Any type of movement can be done in a 30 - 60-minute chunk of time. It might be easier during the week or on busy days to divide your movement into 10-minute segments. One or two 10-minute segments of movement are better than not doing any physical activity at all.

For structured activities, your local city or community usually have programs for adults and children of all ages who want to learn a new sport or participate on competitive or non-competitive teams. These may include soccer, basketball, baseball, tennis, pickleball, volleyball, swimming, gymnastics, or badminton. Dance studios are another place for adults, children, and teens, to get moving. Jazz, hip-hop, ballet, tap dancing, ballroom dancing, salsa dancing, or line dancing anyone? If you belong to a gym, they usually offer a variety of classes and may have some that children or teens can attend, especially in the summer.

Take Action:

There are so many benefits to exercising regularly. If it were a pill, everyone would take it!

Use one or more of the following to get regular exercise:

1. Plan for getting regular exercise. Put it on your calendar and be prepared for your appointment. Have the right attire and shoes, show up on time and think of the benefits.

2. Try several different forms of exercise. Choose the one you like and will do or mix it up for some variety.

3. Get a buddy to exercise with or to have as an accountability partner.

4. Do as recommended by the CDC and walk a total of 150 minutes a week. That's 30 minutes five days a week, 25 minutes 6 days a week, or 21.42 minutes seven days a week. Your choice!

Notes

[1] Why Exercise?
https://www.mayoclinic.org/healthy-lifestyle/fitness/in-depth/exercise/art-20048389

Exercise Fitness Workouts
http://time.com/4474874/exercise-fitness-workouts/

[2] Exercise Recommendations for Children from the CDC
https://www.cdc.gov/physicalactivity/basics/children/index.htm

Exercise Recommendations for Adults from the CDC
https://www.cdc.gov/physicalactivity/basics/adults/index.htm

[3] Exercise Changes Brain: Improve Memory and Thinking Skills
https://www.health.harvard.edu/blog/regular-exercise-changes-brain-improve-memory-thinking-skills-201404097110

You Can Grow New Brain
Cellshttps://www.health.harvard.edu/mind-and-mood/can-you-grow-new-brain-cells

Exercise May Boost the Brain
https://well.blogs.nytimes.com/2013/04/10/how-exercise-may-boost-the-brain

Running and Memory Cell Growth
https://www.theguardian.com/science/2010/jan/18/running-brain-memory-cell-growth

[4] Children Learn Better with Daily Physical
activityhttps://www.parentingscience.com/exercise-for-children.html

Exercise Helps Children Learn Say Experts
https://www.theguardian.com/society/2016/jun/27/exercise-helps-children-learn-say-experts

Exercise Improves
Learninghttp://www.schoolsforchildreninc.org/notebook/study-exercise-improves-learning

CHAPTER 11

Options You May Not Have Considered

Have you ever thought of doing a 5K, 10k, half-marathon, or full marathon? During my sabbatical from work in 2005, when I was recovering from burnout, I received a postcard in the mail from the Stroke Association, a division of the American Heart Association, to participate in a marathon. I was so drawn to it that I had to check it out by attending a meeting about it. At this meeting, I listened to two women, Betty and Sandy, share their inspiring stories. Betty was an 82-year-old stroke and breast cancer survivor. Sandy had a severe stroke while on a business trip and ended up spending a month in rehab before she could fly home. Both women showed off their medals and enthusiastically spoke about completing the full marathon. Inspired, I thought, "if they can do it, so can I." I knew I could downgrade to half-marathon if I needed to. I signed up, raised money, and trained with a group, and in 2006 I completed the 26.2 miles by running and walking and running and walking.

As I trained for the race, I discovered I was capable of doing so much more than I imagined I could do. I was in awe the first time I ran 3 miles, and it felt good! I Never thought I could do that! If you like to walk or run, consider joining a team or training group. Did you know that a large percentage of people completing a half marathon walk them, and a half marathon is the most popular distance of races in the United States?

Training for and participating in a half marathon is one way of getting regular physical activity. I enjoyed being part of a group and went on to become a team captain, leading two groups to raise money and complete their first half marathons. I had to show up! People were counting on me to be there for them. It was a fun and enjoyable way to spend time on weekends.

As covered in the previous chapter, you don't have to do a marathon or a half marathon to get the health benefits of exercise. You can start with a 5K (3.1 miles), or a 10K (6.2 miles), and if you enjoy it, work up to a half marathon (13.1 miles) or a full marathon (26.2 miles). Search online for races in your area, contact charity organizations, or visit a local running store. They may have a training program you can participate in. You can also find training schedules online.

Schedule a Weekend Date with Your Inner Athlete

Do your plans for the weekend include some physical activity? Creating a regular routine on a Saturday or Sunday, morning, afternoon, or evening, may help you attain the health benefits of exercise, and the discipline and motivation to continue with shorter routines during the week.

The benefits of scheduling time on the weekend are:

1. Most people have an hour or two or more for an extra-long walk, run, hike, bike ride, swim, workout, or class at a gym. It allows more time to do activities you may not have the time for during the week.

2. It gives you a chance to participate in a variety of activities that may not be offered during the week.

3. It's easier to find a buddy or a group to exercise with or participate on an adult athletic team through your community parks and recreation.

4. Depending on the ages of your children, the whole family can participate in something together at a park, going bike riding or swimming.

One word of caution, please be mindful of becoming a weekend warrior. Watch that you don't overdo it on the weekend. Participate in some physical activity during the week as well. Your inner athlete will thank you!

Entertainment for Long Walks or Runs

Whether you are training for a race, out on a daily walk, on a treadmill, or a trail, here are some ideas to keep you entertained:

- Use one of the following mantras: "I can, I will, I'm able." "My body is healthy and strong." "Peace, love, joy, well-being, and abundance," or make up your own. Say them or sing them, in your head or out loud, at a slow pace or a fast pace.

- Pay attention to your breathing, your steps or specific body parts and how they move (arms, shoulders, shoulder blades, hips, or feet).

- Send appreciation to your body starting at the top with your head: eyes, ears, nose, mouth, brain, gums, teeth, jaw, throat, shoulders, shoulder blades, lungs, heart, liver, kidneys, spleen, back, arms, hands, elbows, wrists, fingers, digestive system, stomach, intestines, rib cage, hips, legs, knees, shins, calves, feet, ankles, toes, muscles, bones, skin, tendons, immune system, all body systems. You get the idea. See how many parts of your body you can thank for working well.

- Sing some of your favorite songs in your head or out-loud or sing "99 Bottles of Beer on the Wall," forwards and backward. This takes some mental concentration and is fun to do with another person. It's a good distraction for a mile or two!

- List things and people you are grateful for with detail: For example, "I am grateful for my body for functioning so well that I can train for a half marathon (or other distance)." "I am grateful for where I live and enjoy the beauty and peacefulness of nature." "I appreciate my friends who make me laugh." "I'm grateful to have family that loves and supports me." "I appreciate my dog who is adorable and provides unconditional love."

- Play "A to Z games" with a buddy or by yourself, naming things that start with the first letter of the alphabet, then the second letter, and so on. Use categories of foods, states, countries, cities, street names, first names for boys or girls, song titles, companies or brands, etc.

- Visualize yourself being surrounded by light or love or send light or love to a specific area of your body and see if you don't feel lighter and able to move with greater ease.

- Think of as many things as you can that make you happy. "Sunshine, the color red, putting my feet in the sand at the beach, fall leaves, having lunch with a friend, doing puzzles, playing board games..." These are some of what makes me happy!

- If you enjoy listening to music while walking or running, select songs with a slower beat for your warm-up, and songs with a faster beat to help you maintain a quicker workout pace, then back to a slower beat for your cool-down. You can find websites with how to calculate or get song beats per minute for your playlist.[1]

Cold Weather and Physical Activity

As the weather gets colder, do you feel like hibernating? It's easy to look outside and decide that it's too dark out or too cold out to leave your home, let alone go out and exercise.

If you are someone who doesn't like winter weather, you may choose to workout at home to a video or with your own equipment: weights, an exercise bicycle, a treadmill, rowing machine, or mini-trampoline.

For those who feel invigorated by the cold weather, the proper clothing and accessories can make all the difference in being comfortable. Dress in layers of breathable material (wicking clothes and socks), wear a hat to keep your body heat in, gloves to keep your hands warm, and a breathable jacket designed for your specific weather (cold, freezing temperatures, rain, or snow).

How to be Active While Traveling or on Vacation

Traveling for work or fun takes you out of your routine. Getting away can allow for more time to do what you like, reducing your everyday stress level, or it can be hectic and elevate your level of stress.

My number one rule when traveling is to surrender to the process of getting to your destination. Accept that there will be lines of people or lines of cars and delays that are out of your control. Whether you are driving or flying, arriving at an unfamiliar area can be stressful when you don't know your way around.

If you have a delay at an airport, take a walk around to reduce stress, or to get some movement in before your flight. On long drives, take stretch breaks every two hours, and if you can, find a place to walk for 10 minutes. It will refresh you to continue your drive.

Once at your destination, if you haven't done so already, check to see what your options are for physical activity. Many hotels and resorts have a gym included or for an additional charge. An indoor gym is great if the weather outside isn't. Some places offer classes: yoga, Pilates, water aerobics, etc., and may have tennis courts.

Some of the best physical activity is free, like walking on the beach or a self-guided walking tour of an historic area. Playing in the ocean waves, swimming in the pool, or playing water volleyball or catch with your kids can be great ways to bond. There is always the option of taking the stairs rather than the elevator, and lastly, for a strength workout, it's easy to travel with resistance bands.

Plan an Active Vacation

Do you like to hike, bike, walk, run, kayak, or swim? There are vacation destinations that will provide hours of physical activity for you and your family. Consider a hotel with a pool, a water park destination, backpacking, river rafting, walking tours, or participating in a race (5k, 10k, half marathon or full marathon) as a runner or walker.

Keep the following in mind when planning an active vacation:

1. The ages, abilities, and skill level of those going and what is realistic for each person.

2. Equipment and attire, for example, proper shoes (running shoes, hiking boots, sturdy walking shoes, water shoes) and clothing (shorts, swimsuit).

3. Check ahead of time to verify what is included at the site or tour; equipment, meals, lockers, rental fees. Are there package deals, guided tours, or group tours? What are the hours? Is there a minimum age, minimum height, any weight limits, and any health limitations or risks? You'll want to stay hydrated, so make sure to ask about the availability of water and if there is a charge, especially if

you're in a foreign country. I suggest you bring a water bottle when possible.

Take Action:

Never in my wildest dreams did I ever think I would complete a marathon. It wasn't on my radar. It was one of those defining moments that set me on a path I couldn't have planned. There are many ways to move your body that you may not have thought of, both at home and while away on vacation.

Do one or more of the following to make getting regular exercise more enjoyable at home and away.

1. Try something new. Take up a new sport, travel a new route by bike or on foot, do something you've always wanted to do.

2. Discover what's available in your community to participate in for regular exercise.

3. Consider training for a race.

4. Get out for longer stretches of exercise on the weekends.

5. Review the many ways to entertain yourself while exercising to keep your mind busy (on page 111).

6. Plan an active vacation.

Notes

[1] Song Beats per Minute
https://songbpm.com

Beats per Minute Calculator
http://www.beatsperminuteonline.com

How to Build the Ultimate Beats per Minute Playlist
https://lifehacker.com/5646941/how-to-build-the-ultimate-beats-per-minute-optimized-running-playlist

Part Five: Healthy Eating

CHAPTER 12

Finding Your Way Back to Health

Did you know that you can prevent or reverse most food-related diseases and symptoms? I am living proof of this! When I was 19 and had my first blood test, I learned that I had extremely high cholesterol. I was in so much fear of suffering like my mom who had numerous health problems, including off-the-charts cholesterol before she died at 37 years old. Desperate to survive, I made some changes to my diet and added some exercise. A miracle happened! Six weeks later, my follow-up blood test showed that my cholesterol was NORMAL! That was almost four decades ago.

I felt empowered to have control over my health since I didn't trust doctors. They didn't help my mom get well while she suffered from arthritis and migraine headaches, and they didn't save her from breast cancer. After she died, I knew I had to take control of my health. I went to health conventions, read books on nutrition, and even considered becoming a nutritionist. I knew there was a connection between what you eat and illness long before studies proved it to be true.

If you are suffering from heart disease, diabetes, high blood pressure, high cholesterol, high triglycerides, acid reflux, chronic pain, sleep apnea, have had a stroke or cancer, you may benefit significantly by making some changes to what you eat, along with getting some movement to aid in improving blood flow and circulation.[1] The goal is to not be on a "diet," or follow a rigid exercise regime, but rather to create a lifestyle that is sustainable and becomes your way of eating and moving.

Start from Where You Are

How are you? How's your health? Do you know what's going on inside of you? How long has it been since you have had a physical and blood test to see how you are doing on the inside? Even if you're feeling pretty good, it's a good idea to get a baseline of how your body is functioning. A blood test and a check of your blood pressure will give you an assessment of your risk factors for chronic diseases that may be preventable or reversible. If you have chronic stress or chronic pain, need to lose some weight, have high cholesterol, high triglycerides, or high blood pressure, you most likely will be able to improve your health by making some lifestyle changes.

Once you get your baseline information, start from where you are and be realistic about making changes. Remember, you didn't become unhealthy overnight. Be kind to yourself as you decide to make some shifts in your lifestyle. You don't have to go all out or be perfect. Small changes will make a difference. These changes may be in the areas of eating healthier, adding regular physical movement, finding ways to reduce stress and relax, and releasing stored emotions.

If you're under medical care, continue to work with your doctor as you make healthy lifestyle changes. At some point, as you become healthier, you may need to talk about adjusting or eliminating medications, if you are on any.

Transitioning to a Healthy Lifestyle of Eating

Changing to a lifestyle of healthy eating can seem daunting. Committing to make that shift, gradually and sensibly, will give you lasting changes and optimal health.

Start by selecting what seems doable to you. Follow your instincts when something piques your interest. You are the best at knowing what's right for you and what you will or will not eat or drink.

Be willing to trying something new because you WILL have to do something different, on purpose, if you want a different result. Don't worry what you might give up. You don't have to decide to give up anything right now. Keep it easy. Once you start experiencing the benefits of feeling better, having more energy and looking better, it will be easier to embrace and maintain a healthy lifestyle of eating.

One way to transition to a lifestyle of healthy eating is to gradually add vegetables and fruit to what you already eat.

- At breakfast, include bananas, blueberries, blackberries, strawberries, or raspberries. Add spinach, onions, or bell peppers to eggs or egg whites.

- At lunch have a cup of vegetable soup or a salad with your meal.

- At dinner include an extra serving or two of vegetables.

- In between meals, consider eating a piece of fruit: apple, orange, pear, nectarine or peach, or some raw vegetables: carrots, celery, jicama, red or orange bell pepper, tomatoes or cucumber.

An Apple a Day...

While eating an apple a day may keep the doctor away, one piece of fruit a day won't give you the benefits of eating five or more servings of a variety of vegetables and fruit. Eating five or more portions of produce each day has been shown to significantly reduce rates of heart disease, cancer, gastrointestinal disorders, diabetes, and stroke. Other benefits of eating plenty of vegetables and fruit may include the prevention or reversal of high blood pressure, high cholesterol, high triglycerides, sleep apnea, and aid in obtaining and maintaining a healthy body weight.[2]

Boost Your Immune System

When you take good care of your body, you may be able to ward off germs that are in your environment that impact people with weaker immune systems at a higher rate, leading to colds or flu. By eating five or more servings of fruit and vegetables each day, at least one serving at every meal and snack, you keep your body fueled with vitamins, minerals, antioxidants, and phytonutrients.[3]

Eat vegetables and fruit high in antioxidants, vitamins C, E, and beta-carotene, to boost your immune system. These include sweet potatoes, yams, spinach, kale, broccoli, asparagus, cauliflower, snow peas, peppers (green, red, yellow and orange), carrots, tomatoes, collard greens, chard, pumpkin, avocado, oranges, grapefruit, strawberries, raspberries, blueberries, papaya, apples, kiwi, mangos, and pears.

And the Winner Goes to...Water

Hands down, water wins as the most essential component of your body. Did you know that adult bodies are 50 - 60% water? Your brain is 85% water, muscles are 75% water, your blood is 82% water, your lungs are 90% water, and even your bones are 25% water.

Research has shown that for some people, drinking water when you are dehydrated can relieve body aches and pains, including headaches; it can elevate mood and energy, and even lessen symptoms related to allergies and asthma.[4] It's important to drink water to keep your body hydrated to function properly. Another benefit of drinking water is appetite control. By drinking a glass of water before each meal, you will feel less hungry and as a result, eat fewer calories.

Water, the zero-calorie beverage, cannot be substituted by drinking other drinks that contain caffeine, sugar, sugar substitutes and other chemicals, like coffee, tea, soda, sports drinks, and juices. Drinking water helps maintain the balance of body fluids. The functions of these bodily fluids include digestion, absorption, circulation, the creation of saliva, transportation of nutrients, and maintenance of body temperature.[5]

The amount of water a person needs can vary depending on his or her weight, activity level, climate, and the amount of water contained in the foods you eat. Vegetables, fruit, water-based soups, and other foods made with water have a water content that will keep you hydrated in addition to the water you drink.

I start my day with a glass or two of water. I recommend starting your day off with water too. For a warm drink choose caffeine-free tea or add a squeeze of lemon or fresh chopped ginger to hot water. Drink more water throughout the day when you feel thirsty. The more active you are, the more water you will need.

For variety, flavor your water with a wedge or squeeze of lemon, lime, orange, strawberry, pineapple, apple, peach, nectarine, pineapple, mango, cucumber or a mint leaf.

Would You Eat Healthier If It Made You Feel Happier?

A study in the *Journal of Social Indicators Research* found that people who eat seven portions of fruit and vegetables a day have the highest mental well-being and are the happiest.[6] Real food improves your mood!

Next to breathing, eating well and often enough is necessary for your body. When you get too busy or feel tired, it's easy to choose something quick to eat that may not be very good for the functioning of your brain or your body. The next time you feel tired and think about a "pick-me-up" that includes sugar, caffeine or both, remember that it's a temporary solution and may leave you feeling worse a short time later. A better option would be a piece of fruit or a handful of nuts and seeds.

Brain Research and Nutrition

Science is proving that what you eat affects your brain; cognition, memory, attention, stress, and intelligence. The journals *Nutritional Neuroscience* and *European Journal of Clinical Nutrition* have been studying the effects on children in schools that pay attention to nutrition and cognition.[7] There is a direct correlation in children between what they eat and how the brain functions. Those who eat a diet of fruit, vegetables, lean protein, whole grains, and complex carbohydrates have been shown to perform better at school than those who consume a diet of processed foods and fast food high in fats and sugars.

Brain Food

Researchers at Scripps Memorial Hospital in La Jolla, California, have found that blueberries help protect the brain from oxidative stress in animals, and may reduce the effects of age-related conditions such as Alzheimer's disease or dementia. Studies have also shown that diets rich in blueberries significantly improved both the learning capacity and motor skills of aging rats, making them mentally equivalent to much younger rats.[8]

Blueberries are beneficial whether they are fresh, frozen, or dried. Enjoy them by themselves, in oatmeal, yogurt, a smoothie, or in a salad.

Cruciferous Vegetables and Cancer Protection

Cruciferous vegetables contain phytochemicals known as isothiocyanates and indoles, which appear to have a protective effect against some types of cancer. A study by Vanderbilt-Ingram Cancer Center and the Shanghai Center for Disease Control and Prevention investigators revealed that breast cancer survivors who eat more cruciferous vegetables might have improved survival.[9]

Cruciferous vegetables include broccoli, Brussels sprouts, cauliflower, cabbage, arugula, bok choy, collard greens, kale, mustard greens, rutabaga, turnip greens, radish, and watercress.

See the following recipes using cruciferous vegetables in the recipe section of this book:

Broccoli with Fresh Cooked Tomatoes (p. 208)
Broccoli Cranberry Salad (p. 195)
Cauliflower Salad (p. 198)
Cauliflower Fried Rice (p. 209)
Looks Cooked Raw Kale Salad (p. 196)
Michael's Vegetable Soup (p. 190)
Quinoa, Caramelized Onions and Broccoli (p. 208)

Are You Getting Enough Folic Acid – and Why Should You Care?

Here's why: Folic acid (folate) is a B vitamin that is important for the development of red blood cells that carry oxygen around your body and helps maintain good circulation of blood throughout your body.

The consumption of natural foods high in folic acid is essential in the prevention or reversal of many illnesses including heart disease and depression.[10] When your body gets the nutrients it needs and has good circulation, it can function optimally.

Here is a list of foods that are good sources of folic acid:

1. Vegetables and Fruit: romaine lettuce, spinach, kale, asparagus, green beans, peas, cabbage, parsley, turnip greens, collard greens, mustard greens, beets, broccoli, cauliflower, summer squash, fennel, tomatoes, avocado, strawberries, raspberries, and papaya

2. Beans: pinto beans, black beans, garbanzo beans, navy beans, kidney beans, and lentils

3. Whole Grains: whole wheat, wheat germ, bran, brown rice, oatmeal, whole-grain bread and pasta, and barley

Fiber Promotes Health

Fiber has significant health benefits for adults and children. It promotes regularity, prevents constipation, and can aid in weight loss and maintaining a healthy weight. Fiber has also been shown to prevent some cancers, especially colon and breast cancer. Fiber may help lower the LDL cholesterol (the bad cholesterol) and total cholesterol, therefore reducing the risk of heart disease and stroke. Fiber can also aid in lowering blood sugar, thus helping to better manage diabetes, and possibly prevent diabetes.[11]

A product or food item can be labeled "high fiber" when it contains 5 grams or more per serving of fiber. Fiber-containing foods such as vegetables help provide a feeling of fullness with fewer calories. Dietary fiber is in whole grains, vegetables, fruit, cooked beans, peas, lentils, nuts, and seeds. The American Heart Association recommends 25 grams of fiber per day on a 2,000-calorie diet for adults. For women, under 50 years of age the recommendation is 21 - 25 grams per day, and for men under 50, it's 30 - 38 grams per day.[12]

Here are some foods and their fiber content:

1 cup of cooked oatmeal (4 grams)
1/2 cup cooked peas (4.4 grams)
1 cup cooked black beans (15 grams)
1 cup raspberries (8 grams)

Hungry, Tired, and Angry? What and When Did You Eat Last?

There's a saying, "Never let yourself get too hungry, tired, or angry." Did you know that what you eat can have a direct effect on how you feel hours later? Before we get to what you eat, when you eat makes a difference too. When you go too long without eating you may feel tired and irritable. The risk of not eating often enough is that you won't be at your best, and you won't be pleasant to be around if you're unable to manage yourself and your emotions well because you haven't eaten. There is a reason they call this "hangry." Some people do well with three meals a day, while others need a snack in between meals. If you eat a low-fat diet, you will get hungry more quickly than someone eating a moderate or high-fat diet, and you will need to eat more often.

When you're feeling tired, a "sugar fix" may be your go-to solution. You probably have heard about the "sugar crash," which can happen after consuming something high in sugar. Here is what happens in your body when you eat or drink something high in sugar – your body gets a sudden surge of energy followed by an insulin surge that rapidly drops your blood sugar level. Then about two hours later, you feel hungry, tired and possibly irritable.

To avoid a sugar crash, replace simple carbohydrates and processed foods with whole grains and complex carbohydrates. You will feel better and more satisfied. In the next section, which is about carbohydrates, I have included a list of whole grains and complex carbohydrates.

Don't Hate Carbs, Just Be Smart About Them

Carbohydrates have been given a bad name for good reason. Most of the carbohydrates in the standard American diet are simple carbohydrates. These include refined white flour, white rice, and sugars. Think of all the products made with these ingredients.

Did you know that bread and pasta made with white flour have been stripped of most of its nutrients? When wheat berries are processed into white flour, two out of the three nutrient-rich parts, the bran and the germ, get discarded. Those parts contain the fiber, vitamins (B and E) and nutrients (magnesium, zinc, folic acid, and chromium). Only the starchy endosperm is used.

Brown rice becomes white rice by removing the germ and the inner husk (bran). The grain is then polished, usually using glucose or talc. Processed rice has far less vitamin E, thiamine, riboflavin, niacin, vitamin B6, folacin, potassium, magnesium, iron, and over a dozen other nutrients, and the dietary fiber contained in white rice is about a quarter of the amount in brown rice.

Simple carbohydrates are primarily empty calories that may taste good but leave you unsatisfied and wanting more because your body did not get the nutrients it needs to keep you functioning at optimal health. It's like putting low-octane gasoline in a sports car that performs best on high-octane fuel.

Read the list of ingredients and the Nutrition Facts Label when you purchase food products. You will know if you are getting a nutrient-rich product when you see the words whole grain or whole wheat in bread, cereals, and pasta. Other complex carbohydrates include brown rice, quinoa, barley, couscous, beans, lentils, peas, vegetables, and fruit.

Healthy Eating Includes a Variety of Vegetables and Fruit in a Rainbow of Colors.

There are numerous health benefits to eating a variety of whole foods. Each vegetable and fruit contain hundreds if not thousands of phytonutrients unique to that food, in addition to antioxidants, vitamins, minerals, and fiber. Real food heals your body. It really will make a difference in your health. Take a close look at the list of possibilities:

Apples, artichokes, arugula, asparagus, avocado, bamboo shoots, banana, beets, beet greens, bell peppers (green, yellow, orange and red), berries (blueberries, blackberries, strawberries, raspberries), bok choy, broccoli, Brussels sprouts, butternut squash, cabbage (red and green), cantaloupe, carrots, cauliflower, celery, cherries, chives, collard greens, corn, cucumber, dark green leafy lettuces (baby greens), eggplant, endive, escarole, lemon, garlic, grapes (red and green), green beans, grapefruit (red and pink), honeydew melon, hot peppers, kale, kiwi, leeks, mango, mushrooms, nectarine, onions, oranges, papaya, peach, pears, pea pods, pineapple, potatoes, pumpkin, radish, rutabaga, scallions, snow peas, spaghetti squash, spinach, sprouts, star fruit, string beans, summer squash, sweet potatoes, Swiss chard, tomatoes, turnips, water chestnut, watermelon, winter squash, yams and zucchini.

How many of these vegetables and fruits have you tried? How many do you eat regularly? What are your favorites? What sounds new and exciting to try?

A variety of vegetables and fruit can be eaten cooked or raw, by themselves or in recipes. Many vegetables and fruit can be found fresh, frozen, in a jar or canned. For the freshest produce grow your own or visit a local farmer's market to see what vegetables and fruit are in season.

Take Action:

When I was a kid, carrots with a brown sugar glaze (a packaged frozen product) were my favorite vegetable. I didn't dislike vegetables but wasn't crazy about them. After my mother died, I taught myself to eat more veggies by putting sauce on them and putting them in soups. I discovered that I liked steamed squash, and before I knew it, I was enjoying a variety of vegetables. I didn't have anyone telling me I had to eat my veggies, but I knew I had to do something different to eat healthier.

Choose one or more of the suggested actions to be on your way to becoming healthier:

1. Get a baseline of your health with a physical and a blood test.

2. Make a list of vegetables and fruit to add to what you are already eating and then buy them, prepare them, and eat them with meals and snacks!

3. Eat more whole foods and complex carbohydrates.

4. Make water your drink of choice to stay hydrated throughout the day. Drink a large glass of water before your meals and snacks or sip on water throughout your day. For a hot beverage, consider tea, or hot water with fresh ginger or lemon, if desired.

5. Prepare some recipes from the back of this book to help you start eating healthier. Vegetables can taste very different depending on how they are prepared. Roasted vegetables taste different from steamed vegetables or raw vegetables.

6. Keep a tally of how many servings of vegetables and fruit you eat each day. Aim to increase your intake every week or every month until you are eating five or more servings.

7. Track the number of grams of fiber you eat each day for 3 - 7 days. Slowly increase your fiber intake if needed, until you are consuming 21 - 25 grams a day if you're a woman and 30 - 38 grams per day if you're a man.

8. Use the list of the "Rainbow of Colors Foods" (on page 130) to get some ideas of new foods to try or a variety of foods to eat. Then find some ways to prepare the foods or use them in recipes. The Internet is a great place to see how to cook something specific, or to get a recipe using specific ingredients.

Notes

[1] Food-Related Diseases are Preventable or Reversible
http://www.who.int/dietphysicalactivity/publications/trs916/sum maryen/

Diet and Physical Activity
http://www.who.int/dietphysicalactivity/publications/trs916/en

Food Is Medicine
https://draxe.com/food-is-medicine

Reversing Type 2 Diabetes:
https://well.blogs.nytimes.com/2016/04/18/hope-for-reversing-type-2-diabetes

Radical Diet Can Reverse Type 2 Diabetes New Study Shows
https://www.theguardian.com/society/2017/dec/05/radical-diet-can-reverse-type-2-diabetes-new-study-shows

Halting Heart Disease with a Plant-Based Oil-Free Diet
https://www.health.harvard.edu/heart-health/halt-heart-disease-with-a-plant-based-oil-free-diet-

Can You Reverse Heart Disease?
https://www.webmd.com/heart-disease/features/can-you-reverse-heart-disease#1

Dietary Guidelines for Fat and Cholesterol
https://articles.mercola.com/sites/articles/archive/2015/02/25/new-dietary-guidelines-fat-cholesterol.aspx

A Cure for Cancer Eating
https://www.huffingtonpost.com/kathy-freston/a-cure-for-cancer-eating_b_298282.html

Science Says About Diet and Cancer
https://www.forksoverknives.com/science-says-about-diet-and-cancer

[2] Benefits of Eating 5 or More Servings of Produce
https://www.medicalnewstoday.com/articles/267290.php

An Apple a Day May Not Keep the Doctor Away
https://www.health.harvard.edu/blog/an-apple-a-day-may-not-keep-the-doctor-away-but-its-a-healthy-choice-anyway-201504027850

What Should You Eat? Vegetables and Fruit
https://www.hsph.harvard.edu/nutritionsource/what-should-you-eat/vegetables-and-fruits

Eating More Fruits and Vegetables May Prevent Millions of Premature Deaths
http://www3.imperial.ac.uk/newsandeventspggrp/imperialcollege/newssummary/news_22-2-2017-16-38-0

Six Best Diets for Sleep Apnea
http://www.apneatreatmentcenter.com/6-best-diets-for-sleep-apnea-2017-edition

Lifestyle Modifications and the Resolution of Obstructive Sleep Apnea Syndrome: A Case Report
https://www.ncbi.nlm.nih.gov/pmc/articles/PMC3110415

Diet and Exercise in the Management of Obstructive Sleep Apnea and Cardiovascular Disease Risk
http://err.ersjournals.com/content/26/144/160110

Beating High Blood Pressure with Food
https://www.health.harvard.edu/newsletter_article/beating-high-blood-pressure-with-food

[3] What Are Phytonutrients?
https://www.webmd.com/diet/guide/phytonutrients-faq#1

[4] Health Benefits of Water
https://greatist.com/health/health-benefits-water

Asthma – Is There a Connection Between Dehydration?
https://asthma.net/living/ask-the-experts-is-there-a-connection-between-dehydration/

Seven Health Benefits of Water
https://www.healthline.com/nutrition/7-health-benefits-of-water#section2

What You Should Know About Drinking Water (but Probably Don't)
https://www.nbcnews.com/better/diet-fitness/down-low-h20-n760721

Does Drinking More Water Help with Joint Pain?
https://www.livestrong.com/article/448421-does-drinking-more-water-help-with-joint-pain

[5] Six Reasons to Drink Water
https://www.webmd.com/diet/features/6-reasons-to-drink-water#1

[6] The Connection Between Eating Fruit and Vegetables and Psychological Well-Being
https://www.medicalnewstoday.com/articles/315781.php

Nutritional Psychiatry: Your Brain on Food
https://www.health.harvard.edu/blog/nutritional-psychiatry-your-brain-on-food-201511168626

[7] The Effect of Food and Nutrition on Children's Mental State and Performance
https://pdfs.semanticscholar.org/74d0/c730d77447280f8f6bb5abca1389bc9a965a.pdf

[8] Eat More Berries for Greater Brain Power
https://nutritionallyyourstestkits.com/eat-berries-greater-brain-power

[9] Eating Cruciferous Vegetables May Improve Breast Cancer Survival
https://www.sciencedaily.com/releases/2012/04/120403153531.htm

[10] Folic Acid Preventing and Reversing Illnesses
http://www.heartdiseaseonline.com/aa/aa122798.htm
https://www.ncbi.nlm.nih.gov/pmc/articles/PMC4559887

Vitamin B12 and Folic Acid Improve Memory in Two-year Trial
http://www.lifeextension.com/Newsletter/2011/12/Vitamin-B12-Folic-Acid-Improve-Memory-In-Two-Year-Trial/Page-01

Depression Won't Go Away? Folate Could Be the Answer
https://www.psychologytoday.com/blog/the-integrationist/

[11] Fiber and Weight Control
https://www.webmd.com/diet/features/fiber-weight-control#1

Fiber Can Help with Weight Loss
https://www.health.harvard.edu/blog/making-one-change-getting-fiber-can-help-weight-loss-201502177721

How Fiber Helps Protect Against Cancer
https://www.pcrm.org/health/cancer-resources/diet-cancer/nutrition/how-fiber-helps-protect-against-cancer

Disease Conditions and High Blood Cholesterol
https://www.mayoclinic.org/diseases-conditions/high-blood-cholesterol/in-depth/cholesterol/art-20045192

Cholesterol-Lowering Effects of Dietary Fiber: A Meta-Analysis (1999)
https://www.everydayhealth.com/type-2-diabetes/diet/control-high-blood-sugar-with-fiber

Nutrition and Healthy Eating
https://www.mayoclinic.org/healthy-lifestyle/nutrition-and-healthy-eating/in-depth/fiber/art-20043983

[12] American Heart Association Recommendations for Fiber
http://www.heart.org/HEARTORG/HealthyLiving/HealthyEating/HealthyDietGoals/Whole-Grains-and-Fiber_UCM_303249_Article.jsp#.Wj0ZP1WnGpp

Fiber Supplementation in Obese Individuals Significantly Enhances Weight Loss."
https://www.ncbi.nlm.nih.gov/pubmed/19335713

How Much Fiber Should Children Eat?
https://www.bundoo.com/articles/how-much-fiber-should-children-eat

CHAPTER 13

Are You at Risk?

Diabetes, high blood pressure, and obesity have been diagnosed in adults and children at an alarming rate. So have high cholesterol, high triglycerides, heart disease, sleep apnea, and chronic illnesses. The good news is that these medical conditions are primarily diet related and in most cases are preventable or treatable.

Genetic factors can play a role in childhood and adult obesity and associated health problems. Shared family behaviors tend to play an even more significant role in our health problems. Eating and activity habits are how a "family history of health problems" get passed down from one generation to another. For me, having high cholesterol and struggling to maintain a healthy and comfortable weight was passed down to me because of the types of food I was raised to eat. A diet heavy in meat and dairy created my high cholesterol. Plus, I never saw my parents as active people, so I didn't learn to stay active.

Our childhood associations with food can also contribute to life-long unhealthy eating. Messages about food, emotional eating, and a sedentary lifestyle are the cause of many of the diseases people have today.

Are You Aware of What You Eat?

Do you make it a practice to read Nutrition Fact Labels and ingredient lists on the foods you buy? Do you have an idea of how much unprocessed food you eat in relation to processed food?

Living a lifestyle of healthy eating, that is, eating a diet made up primarily of real food, whole foods, vegetables, fruit, whole grains, beans, lentils, nuts, and seeds, has been shown to provide optimal health. Switching to a plant-based diet, with small amounts of chicken and fish, if you choose, has been shown to prevent and reverse food-related illnesses that so many people suffer from by eating a diet high in fat, cholesterol, sugar, and sodium that come from consuming too much fast food and processed food.[1]

Getting in the habit of reading Nutrition Food Labels will help you understand just how many calories you are consuming along with the breakdown of fats, sugar, cholesterol, sodium, protein, and fiber. When reading the ingredient lists, remember that ingredients are listed in order of highest content to least. Also, keep in mind that there are many names for sugar and a food item will often show more than one form. An example would be a product that uses both honey and agave, with smaller amounts of each than if the product only used one form of sugar. (See page 146 for a list of different names for sugar.) Additionally, be on the lookout for ingredients you can't pronounce or are unfamiliar with. Beware of artificial flavorings, colors, or other man-made chemicals to preserve and make the food taste better.

Healthy and Unhealthy Fats

Unhealthy fats include saturated fat and trans fats. Saturated fats come mostly from animal products such as meat, poultry, and dairy products. The American Heart Association recommends no more than 5% to 6% of total daily calories from saturated fat.[2]

Trans fats, also known as partially hydrogenated oils, are found in many fried foods and baked goods. The FDA concluded that removing partially hydrogenated oils from processed foods could prevent thousands of heart attacks and deaths each year.[3] Most trans fats have been removed from processed foods and fast food chains since the FDA's finding.

Healthier fats are unsaturated fats. These include polyunsaturated and monounsaturated fats. They are found mainly in fish such as salmon, trout, and herring; avocados, olives, walnuts; and liquid vegetable oils such as soybean, corn, safflower, canola, olive, and sunflower. While consuming a small amount of oil is needed for health, keep in mind that oils contain about 120 calories per tablespoon. Therefore, the amount of oil consumed needs to be limited to balance your total calorie intake. The Nutrition Facts Label on food products provides information to help you make wise choices.

Omega-3 and Omega-6 Fatty Acids

Omega-3 and omega-6 fatty acids are considered essential fatty acids: They are necessary for your health, and your body can't make them. You must get them through food. Omega-3 fatty acids can be found in fish, such as salmon, tuna, halibut, and other seafood including algae and krill, and some plants and nut oils. Both omega-3 and omega-6 fatty acids play a crucial role in brain function as well as normal growth and development and may also reduce the risk of heart disease.

Omega-6 fatty acids, also known as polyunsaturated fatty acids (see Healthy and Unhealthy Fats section on the previous page), help stimulate skin and hair growth, maintain bone health, regulate metabolism, and maintain the reproductive system.

A healthy diet contains a balance of omega-3 and omega-6 fatty acids. Omega-3 fatty acids help reduce inflammation, while some omega-6 fatty acids may promote inflammation. The typical American diet tends to contain 14 or more times the amount of omega-6 fatty acids than omega-3 fatty acids. The bad news is that we get too much omega-6 fatty acids and not nearly enough omega-3 fatty acids. This imbalance is responsible for numerous chronic health disorders including a rise in blood pressure that can lead to blood clots that can cause heart attack and stroke, and cause your body to retain water.[4] A lower ratio of omega-6 to omega-3 fatty acids is more desirable in reducing the risk of many of the chronic diseases of high prevalence in Western societies.[5]

What Is Cholesterol and Where Is it Found?

Cholesterol is a waxy, fatty substance that travels through your bloodstream. Your body needs cholesterol to build cells and produce certain hormones. Your body produces all the cholesterol it needs in the liver and intestines from the foods you eat, namely fats, sugars, and proteins.

Cholesterol is also in animal products and dairy products: meat, fish, chicken, turkey, pork, butter, milk, eggs, yogurt, cheese, and ice cream. When you consume too many saturated and trans fats, it causes your liver to produce too much "bad" cholesterol, which winds up clogging your arteries. Having a higher level of cholesterol is a risk factor for heart disease. It is recommended to limit saturated fats to 10% or less of your total caloric intake.[6]

Sodium

Packaged foods and beverages can contain high levels of sodium, whether or not they taste salty. A diet high in sodium draws water into the bloodstream, which can increase the volume of blood and subsequently your blood pressure. High blood pressure or hypertension is a condition in which blood pressure remains elevated over time. Hypertension makes the heart work harder, and the high force of the blood flow can harm arteries and organs (such as the heart, kidneys, brain, and eyes). Eating less sodium can help lower blood pressure, which in turn, can help reduce your risk of developing dangerous medical conditions.

Check the Nutrition Facts Label on products to find out how much sodium is in a serving. The daily recommendation for sodium, according to the FDA, is less than 2,400 milligrams (mg) per day.[7]

The Lowdown on Sugar

Why does sugar have to taste so good and not be good for you? Before the invention of processed food, when people ate what nature provided, people believed that if something tasted sweet, it was safe to eat. While this may have kept humans alive centuries ago, today it is creating quite a health crisis.

Excessive sugar intake can cause significant weight gain, lead to type 2 diabetes, and heart disease.[8] The empty calories in sugar don't provide any nutritional benefit, often leaving you feeling unsatisfied and wanting to eat more.

How Are Americans Consuming Over 100 Pounds of Sugar a Year?

Today, the average American consumes over 100 pounds of sugar a year, not including naturally occurring sugars in milk, fruit, and vegetables.[9]

Where is all that sugar coming from? Sugars and syrups are being added to almost every category of food and drink during processing or preparation. Foods that contain the most added sugar are:

- Regular soft drinks
- Candy
- Cakes
- Cookies
- Pies
- Fruit drinks, fruit punch, and sweetened beverages
- Bread products: sweet rolls and cinnamon toast
- Milk-based desserts and products: ice cream, sweetened yogurt, and sweetened milk, like chocolate milk

Sugar is also in these "not so obvious" foods and condiments:

- Salad Dressing
- Bread
- Stuffing Mix
- Soups
- Ketchup
- Crackers
- Barbecue Sauce
- Macaroni and Cheese
- Hamburger Buns
- Pasta Sauce
- Breakfast Cereals
- Yogurt
- Teriyaki Sauce
- Juice Drinks

How Much Sugar Is Recommended to Eat?

The American Heart Association advises:[10]

- Women to have no more than six teaspoons, 25 grams, or 100 calories from sugar per day, and

- Men to have no more than nine teaspoons, 36 grams, or 150 calories from sugar per day.

That's just over 20 pounds of sugar per year for women and almost 29 pounds of sugar per year for men.

There are four calories in one gram of sugar, so if a product has 15 grams of sugar per serving, **that's 60 calories just from the sugar alone, not counting the other ingredients.**

Are You Up for a Challenge?

Put on your detective hat and get out your magnifying glass. Here is your mission. Look for different names for sugar on the ingredient list of foods and beverages at your home or a market. Then check the number of grams of sugar on the Nutrition Facts Label. Remember to also look at how much is a serving. It might surprise you to see how much sugar you are consuming!

These are all names for sugar:

agave nectar, apple juice, barley malt, beet sugar, brown rice syrup, brown sugar, buttered syrup, carob syrup, castor sugar, confectioner's sugar, cane crystals, cane sugar, caramel, corn sweetener, corn syrup, crystalline fructose, fruit juice concentrate, date sugar, dehydrated cane juice, demerara sugar, dextran, dextrose, diatase, diatatic malt, ethyl maltol, fructo-oligosaccharides, evaporated cane juice, fruit juice, fruit juice concentrate, galactose, glucose, glucose solids, golden syrup, fructose, granulated sugar, grape juice, grape sugar, high fructose corn syrup, honey, invert sugar, lactose, malted barley, maltitol, maltodextrin, maltose, malt syrup, mannitol, maple sugar, maple syrup, microcrystalline cellulose, molasses, organic dehydrated cane sugar, muscovado sugar, pear juice, polydextrose, powdered sugar, raisin juice, raw sugar, refiner's syrup, rice syrup, saccharose, sorbitol, sorghum, sorghum syrup, sucanat, sucrose, sugar, sugar

cane, syrup, treacle, turbinado sugar, vanilla sugar, white grape juice, white sugar, xylitol, xylose, yellow sugar

---

Sugar Alcohols

Sugar alcohols commonly found in foods are sorbitol, mannitol, xylitol, isomalt, and hydrogenated starch hydrolysates. Sugar alcohols come from plant products such as fruits and berries. The carbohydrates in these plant products are altered through a chemical process. These sugar substitutes provide somewhat fewer calories than table sugar (sucrose), mainly because they are not well absorbed and may even have a small laxative effect.[11]

Though the word "alcohol" is part of their name, they cannot get you drunk. And because they are not completely absorbed, they can ferment in the intestines and cause bloating, gas, or even diarrhea. People can have different individual reactions to different sugar alcohols. Careful experimentation is advised.[12]

Look at What a Serving Is

With the significant increase in the amount of food that people have been eating since the 1970s, you might be confused about what a serving size is. Here is a fun way to look at serving sizes:

Meat, fish or poultry (3 oz.) = a deck of cards

Rice or pasta (1 cup) = a tennis ball

1 potato (white or sweet) = a computer mouse

1/2 cup cooked vegetables = a baseball

1 oz. bread, toast or 1 pancake = a CD case

1/4 cup nuts or dried fruit = a golf ball

1 tablespoon peanut butter = a Ping-Pong ball

1 oz. hard cheese = 4 dice

1 teaspoon oil = a water-bottle cap

Activity: Get out your measuring cups; 1/4 cup, 1/2 cup, and 1 cup. Measure out the suggested food items below or substitute other items with similar serving sizes. (See the Nutrition Facts Label for serving sizes on packaged foods.) Then put the food item in a bowl or on a plate so you can see what a serving size looks like displayed to eat.

1/4 cup almonds
1/2 cup cooked vegetables
1 cup cooked pasta

Take a good look at what a serving is. Are you surprised?

Remember to look closely at the serving size. Food companies sometimes have different serving sizes for the same product. For example, on a loaf of bread, one company may list one slice of bread as a serving while another has two slices as a serving.

Take Action:

You can take the guesswork out of what to eat and how much to eat when you are mindful of your options and portions.

Become aware of what you eat by doing one or more of the following:

1. Make a habit of reading food labels for ingredients, serving size, and nutrition facts.

2. Go on a hunt for the many names of sugar listed on ingredient labels (see page 146).

3. Track how many grams of sugar you eat each day for 3 - 7 days, excluding naturally occurring sugars in milk, fruit, and vegetables.

4. See what a serving size is by measuring out a few different foods (on page 148). Use smaller dishes and bowls if the quantity of food appears too small for you. Yes, it is a mind thing, and it will make a difference.

Notes

[1] Benefits of a Plant-Based Diet
(See Chapter 12 - Finding Your Way Back to Health, on page 119.)

[2] The Skinny on Fats
http://www.heart.org/HEARTORG/Conditions/Cholesterol/PreventionTreatmentofHighCholesterol/The-Skinny-on-Fats_UCM_305628_Article.jsp#.WouMgIPwapo

[3]Healthy and Unhealthy Fats
https://www.fda.gov/Food/IngredientsPackagingLabeling/FoodAdditivesIngredients/ucm449162.htm

[4] The Truth About Fats
https://www.webmd.com/women/features/benefits-of-essential-fats-and-oils#1

[5] Omega-3 and Omega-6 Fatty Acids
https://www.ncbi.nlm.nih.gov/pubmed/12442909

[6] High Cholesterol
https://www.healthline.com/health/high-cholesterol/rda

[7] Sodium
https://www.fda.gov/Food/ResourcesForYou/Consumers/ucm315393.htm

[8] Sugar Increases the Risk of Dying with Heart Disease
https://www.health.harvard.edu/blog/eating-too-much-added-sugar-increases-the-risk-of-dying-with-heart-disease-201402067021

[9] The Average American Consumes 150 - 170 Pounds of Sugar Each Year
https://bamboocorefitness.com/not-so-sweet-the-average-american-consumes-150-170-pounds-of-sugar-each-year

---

[10] American Heart Association Recommendations on Sugar http://www.heart.org/HEARTORG/HealthyLiving/HealthyEating/Nutrition/Added-Sugars_UCM_305858_Article.jsp#

[11] What Are Sugar Alcohols?
https://www.joslin.org/info/what_are_sugar_alcohols.html

[12] How Sugar Alcohols Can Impact Your Health
https://www.verywellfit.com/what-are-sugar-alcohols-2242525

CHAPTER 14

Could You Spend $2,000 Every Day?

If you were given $2,000 every day, you might have a challenging time spending that much money, every single day. If you were given $2,000 a day and you had to buy your calories at $1/calorie, you might easily spend that much before noon, or on one meal!

Are you ready to have some fun? My family played this game that I created when our children were young, and I wanted to teach them about eating with awareness.

Calories are your body's energy currency. Calories are used to create energy for your body's daily activities. Olympic athletes can fuel their bodies with 5,000 or more calories each day, while most of us non-professional athletes only need a fraction of that, about 1600 – 2500 calories a day. (Check with your doctor to determine your ideal weight and caloric needs.) The more active you are, the more energy your body needs.

This chapter is the Activity: Make it a game and try this on your own or with your family: "Buy" your calories for three days in a row and see how much you are really "spending." You don't need real cash to do this. Money from games like Monopoly or Payday will work, or you can make your own currency. Include EVERYTHING you eat, drink, and chew. That's everything you have for breakfast, lunch, dinner, all drinks, snacks, tastes, candies, and gum.

For calorie information, see the Nutrition Facts Label of each food item for calories per serving and serving size. When eating out, the calories may be posted on the menu. If those options are unavailable, there are many sites online that have calorie count information.

No matter what "diet" you choose, your body needs calories for energy, and unused calories get stored as fat. Eat with awareness. It will help you make better choices for a healthier body.

Take Action:

This game is a chapter in itself. I wanted it to stand out!

Here's how to play:

1. Determine your ideal weight and caloric needs. Based on how many calories you need, you will give yourself that much "money" each day to spend on calories at a dollar per calorie.

2. Gather some board game money or make your own currency to play the $2,000 a day game. Put your allotted money for the day in an envelope.

3. Keep a log of what you eat and drink, and the calorie count for the portions for three days.

4. After each meal or snack, pay for your calories with your money.

5. At the end of each day, look over your log and answer the following questions:

6. Were you surprised to see how fast your money went?

7. Are you more aware of what you are eating and how much of it?

8. Did you modify your eating habits because you are playing this game and didn't want to spend your calories on a food or beverage?

9. What will you do different tomorrow, if anything?

10. Repeat the above steps for days 2 and 3.

CHAPTER 15

Dozens of Ways to Healthier Eating

It wasn't always easy for me to eat healthy, especially when I was first starting. I was in my third year of college at USC, highly stressed, and not sure I could survive and get through the rigorous and highly competitive business school. I was living at home with an hour-long commute, and I had a daily habit of buying a huge oatmeal cookie for my drive home.

I decided I was ready to lose some weight and saw an advertisement in the newspaper for the Pritikin Program[1]. It was through that program that I had my first blood test, learned of having extremely high cholesterol, and lowered it with healthy eating.

I've used what I've learned over time and have taken the guesswork out of eating healthier, and now I'm sharing it with you! This chapter is packed with practical ways to eat healthy while at home and away.

You can eat healthier at every meal and snack when you know in advance what to eat. As you read this chapter, see yourself planning, making a list, knowing when you will go grocery shopping, and when you will do some food prep and cooking.

Time for Breakfast

We've all heard that breakfast is supposed to be the most important meal of the day, but do you know why? A healthy breakfast fuels your body with calories so that it can function. It provides needed nutrients, especially phytonutrients from fruit and vegetables. Also, eating breakfast can help boost your metabolism, and that may help with weight loss and weight control.

Plan your morning so that you have time to eat breakfast. For example, I often have oatmeal, so I'll take out the oats, a bowl, a spoon, and a measuring cup the night before. Then in the morning, I don't have to go looking in the cupboards and drawers for these items. All I need to do is cook the oatmeal and add sliced banana or some blueberries and walnuts or chia seeds and cinnamon. (See Oatmeal Recipe Ideas on page 182.)

A high fiber (5 grams per serving), low sugar (5 - 7 grams per serving) breakfast cereal is another option. Add low-fat milk, or an almond or soy beverage and fruit for a satisfying, healthy breakfast. If you eat dairy, add fruit and a tablespoonful of walnuts or almonds to plain yogurt.

Breakfast can consist of any whole grain leftovers like quinoa or brown rice and vegetables, or an omelet with leftover vegetables and a side of cooked beans. You could even have soup for breakfast or a salad.

Just as with other meals, a healthy breakfast will have a combination of some of these: vegetables, fruit, whole grains, lean protein, nuts, seeds, lentils, and legumes.

What's for Lunch?

People who pack their lunches have more control over what they eat, tend to eat healthier, and save money at the same time. Dining on a pre-packed lunch can aid in weight loss and weight management.

The following are some lunch ideas and recipes. There are more recipes included at the back of the book:

- Make a salad. Start with lettuce, spinach, or kale. Add a serving or two of raw or cooked vegetables. For protein, add a portion or two of quinoa, almonds, hemp seeds, beans, or lentils. With all of the ingredients in your salad, you may not need any salad dressing, or a drizzle of dressing may be sufficient.

- Almost any leftovers from dinner can make a great lunch: cooked vegetables with brown rice, whole grain pasta, lentils, quinoa, precooked chicken or salmon, baked yam or sweet potato, soup, etc.

- Add some fruit to your lunch: apple, banana, pear, grapes, orange, berries, etc., or make a fruit salad.

- For a light lunch, have raw vegetables: carrots, celery, jicama, red peppers, peapods, broccoli, cauliflower with hummus. (See recipe for Easy Homemade Hummus on page 188.)

Here are a variety of flavorful salad recipes:

Black Bean Salad (p. 197)
Looks Cooked Raw Kale Salad (p. 196)
Broccoli Cranberry Salad (p. 195)
Cauliflower Salad (p. 198)

Here are more recipes:

Zucchini Rice Bake (p. 206)
Lentils with Broccoli and Pasta Sauce (p. 200)
Quinoa, Caramelized Onions, and Broccoli (p. 208)
Celery Barley Soup (p. 193)
Rice, Beans and Tomato (p. 201)

If you don't already pack a lunch, try it once or twice a week. You just might get into the habit of it! An easy way to get started is to make an extra serving or two of something you are already going to make, then pack your lunch when you are putting the extra food into storage containers. Your lunch will be ready to go in the morning when you pre-plan and pre-package your food the night before and save you time too.

Dinner's On!

Anything that you would eat for breakfast or lunch would make a great dinner! Follow the guidelines from the prior two sections, "Time for Breakfast" and "What's for Lunch?" Some people like to eat a more substantial lunch and a smaller dinner or vice versa. What matters most is that you feel satisfied! See the "Main Dish" recipes (starting on page 199) at the back of this book for more options.

Let's Get You on Your Way to Eating Healthy

It can be difficult to want to eat healthier and not have the habits developed yet, so here are some suggestions to get you on your way. Choose ONE or TWO new ways to practice for the next 3 - 7 days. Start from where you are and ease into any changes gradually so that they will become lasting new habits.

1. Decrease portions of unhealthy foods as you develop a new healthy eating lifestyle. For example, if you eat pizza, have one less slice of pizza than usual. If you tend to eat large or second servings of high-fat or high-sugar foods, cut your portions in half.

2. Add vegetables to what you already eat. Have raw vegetables washed, cut into pieces, and ready to eat in the refrigerator. They will be easy to snack on with a dip like hummus or put into a salad.

3. Have a side salad with lunch or dinner.

4. Plan your snacks, especially when on the go. Have a piece of fruit and a serving of almonds or some raw vegetables.

5. Eat fresh fruit when you want something sweet, for a snack, or with a meal.

How to Simplify Your Weekly Food Preparation

With a little planning ahead and food preparation, eating healthy meals and snacks is easy! Back when I was 19 years old and chose to change the way I ate to lower my cholesterol, I figured out how to simplify the process of meal planning and preparation by cooking in large quantities then freezing a lot of what I made for meals for the coming days and weeks. Decades later, I still cook in large batches.

Here are some suggestions:

1. Select a few recipes to prepare. I usually choose one or two soups and make a big pot full of each. Once they are cooled, keep some to eat during the week and freeze the rest in labeled containers.

2. Cook multiple servings of quinoa, brown rice, or whole grain pasta. These all will keep in the refrigerator for up to a week or can be frozen.

3. Precook vegetables by steaming, sautéing, baking, or roasting. They will stay good in the refrigerator for 4 - 5 days or can be frozen. A large batch of steamed broccoli can be warmed up as a side dish, added to a soup or served cold on a salad. Baked yams can be eaten right out of their skin as a side dish, in a salad, or even for dessert.

4. Pre-cut raw vegetables for snacking, to put in salads or to take "on the go."

Once you have some vegetables and grains prepared, you can easily combine them to make a quick and easy meal to eat at home or while at work or school. These combinations often taste good eaten hot or cold. Add a salad and some fruit to go with your prepared soup, vegetables, and grains, and you will easily be eating healthy and feeling satisfied.

Healthy "On-The-Go" Snack Ideas

To limit the temptation of buying food when out and about, plan ahead and always carry snacks!

A serving of almonds or whole grain crackers may tide you over until you get home if you are out longer than expected and find yourself getting hungry or just wanting to eat something. Almost anything you make in your kitchen or bring with you is going to be healthier, and lower in fat and calories than what you can get at a fast food restaurant or coffee establishment.

Here are food items that travel well and some tips:

1. Almonds, whole grain crackers, and whole wheat pretzels in single-serving containers, can be kept in your car, a purse or backpack.

2. Most other snacks are perishable and need to be stored in an insulated lunch bag or mini ice chest.

- Whole Fruit: apple, banana, peach, plum, nectarine, apricot, pear, grapes, berries – pack some napkins too!
- Cut-up Fruit: watermelon, cantaloupe, honeydew, or a mini fruit salad; remember to bring a fork!
- Raw Vegetables: carrot sticks, celery sticks, sliced red bell peppers, jicama sticks; and make sure to bring napkins too!
- Dairy: string cheese, yogurt, and a spoon!

3. Water is always an excellent choice for a drink. Sometimes when you feel hungry, you are actually dehydrated, and drinking water may be just what you need instead of food.

What Could Seven Servings of Vegetables and Fruit Look Like?

Breakfast could include one or two servings of vegetables or fruit: potatoes, peppers, onions, spinach, avocado, tomatoes, a banana, 1/2 a grapefruit, an orange, blueberries, blackberries, raspberries, strawberries, grapes, or melon.

A mid-morning and late afternoon snack could contain one serving: an apple, pear, grapes, carrots, snap peas, celery or red bell pepper. Lunch could comprise two or more servings of vegetables: a green salad with raw or cooked vegetables; broccoli, cauliflower, carrots, cabbage, beets, red, orange or yellow bell peppers, celery, or cucumber.

Dinner could include two or more servings of vegetables from any of the following: vegetable soup, a salad, cooked greens, or a medley of vegetables. Try these recipes:

Michael's Vegetable Soup (p. 190)
Delicious Greens with Garlic (p. 209)
Asparagus, Red Peppers, and Onions (p. 212)
Steamed Vegetable Medley (p. 207)

It's easy to add vegetable and fruit servings to what you already eat when you plan ahead! See the recipes in the back of this book for more variety.

Five Ways to Add More Vegetables to Meals

It's easy to create a healthy diet when you focus on adding more vegetables to what you already eat, rather than on what you need to remove.

1. Plan meals around a main vegetable dish, such as a vegetable stir-fry, ratatouille, or vegetable soup. Then add other foods to complement it. These can include brown rice, quinoa, a baked potato or yam, a side of beans or lentils, or a small serving (about 2 ounces) of lean meat, chicken, or fish.

2. Have a green salad with your dinner every night. Add raw vegetables, such as carrots, celery, red, orange or yellow bell peppers, tomatoes, cauliflower, jicama, peas, cucumber, broccoli, radish, or artichoke hearts.

3. Include chopped vegetables in pasta sauce: zucchini, broccoli, eggplant, carrots, spinach, onions, peppers, or fresh tomatoes.

4. Use pureed cooked vegetables such as potatoes, zucchini, onions, and carrots to thicken stews, soups, and gravies. These add flavor, nutrients, and texture.

5. Grill vegetable kabobs as part of a barbecue meal. Try cherry or grape tomatoes, mushrooms, zucchini, onions, summer squash, yellow squash, or red, orange, yellow, or green peppers.

Vegetable of the Week

While it is wise to eat a wide variety of vegetables, it is cost effective to build meals around fresh, seasonal, reasonably priced produce. By selecting one or two primary vegetables, it allows you to prepare a larger quantity to use for multiple meals.

Here are some examples using broccoli:

1. Steam, stir-fry, or cook several servings of broccoli briefly in boiling water.

2. Use the cooked vegetable as a side dish, on salads, with brown rice, quinoa, lentils, or whole grain pasta. Add to store-bought soups or make a quick soup with broth, the precooked vegetable, and brown rice or quinoa. Precooked vegetables can also be used to create an omelet or homemade burritos or quesadillas.

3. Use broccoli in the following recipes:

Leftovers Soup (p. 191)
Vegetable Stir-Fry (p. 204)
Michael's Vegetable Soup (p. 190)
Broccoli Cranberry Salad (p. 195)
Lentils with Broccoli and Pasta Sauce (p. 200)
Quinoa, Caramelized Onions, and Broccoli (p. 208)

Greens, Greens, Greens!

Greens have been touted as some of the healthiest foods available. Some people love them, while others don't care for them, or rather, they haven't found a way to prepare them that is enjoyable.

The "greens" food group includes spinach, kale, arugula, bok choy, beet greens, chard, collard greens, and mustard greens, among others.

Arugula is a "green" that has been classified as a "Superfood." At only 16 calories per two-cup serving, it is packed with nutrients, including vitamin A (great for your eyes and vision) and Vitamin K (known for bone- building). Mature arugula has a spicier, peppery taste, while baby arugula has a milder flavor with the same health benefits.

Here are some ways to enjoy arugula, or any other leafy green:

1. Make a salad with a variety of greens.

2. Add arugula leaves to a sandwich.

3. Sauté greens in a small amount of olive oil and serve as a side dish, or add to cooked quinoa, brown rice, or whole grain pasta.

4. Add greens to vegetable or lentil soup.

5. Place arugula, spinach, or kale leaves on a pizza before baking.

You'll find the following recipes at the back of the book for three very different ways of preparing greens:

Delicious Greens with Garlic (p. 209)
Looks Cooked Raw Kale Salad (p. 196)
Nourishing Power Smoothie (p. 185)

Sweets

The next time you are craving something sweet, have a piece of fruit. Sweet summer fruits; peaches, nectarines, watermelon, berries, kiwi, melons, plums, cherries, apricots, etc. Okay, they may not always satisfy that craving, but I think this is what nature intended in the sweets department. By adding one or two servings of fruit to your daily eating, you can change your taste buds over time, and one day you may find that your cravings for sweets will be satisfied by fruit.

What's the Buzz about Juicing?

Juicing is a process that extracts the juices from whole fruits and vegetables. People substitute "juice" for eating the whole food to get the benefit of bio-available nutrients to their cells without the need of their body to break down food or fiber, making the vitamins, minerals, enzymes, and phytonutrients easy to absorb in quantities that could never be consumed. (See Juicing Tips and Recipes on page 186.)

I have personally seen the benefits of juicing in three people I want to highlight. One used juicing to get healthy and lose weight, and as a result, he was able to get off high blood pressure medication and eliminate the need to use a sleep apnea machine. Another used juicing while going through radiation treatment after cancer surgery. She expressed having more energy, and overall feeling healthier when she drinks juiced vegetables. The third person eliminated the pain in her hands that she had previously accepted as "normal" aging.

Too Much of a Good Thing

"If a little is good, more is better." Many people believe in this motto, especially when it comes to eating healthy food. Consuming a lot of one particular food or food group can cause two potential problems. One, you may be depriving your body of necessary nutrients; and two, you may end up eating too many or too few calories.

Here are two examples:

1. We can all agree that kale and spinach are healthy foods. If most of your diet were made up of these two greens, you would not be taking in enough calories or nutrients.

2. Eating excessive servings of dried fruit, nuts, and seeds (almonds, walnuts, sunflower seeds, etc.), avocado, or whole grains will lead to an excess of calories and weight gain and may leave you too full for other nutritious foods.

Everything in moderation!

Involve Your Friends and Family

A potluck dinner is a great way to bring people together who have an interest in eating healthier, trying new recipes, and having fun doing it! Several years ago, I started a "Healthy Potluck" dinner club that met monthly at different homes.

All it takes is contacting some friends and family, and sending out an email invitation to 6 - 8 people or more to get together and enjoy some new healthy foods!

Here is a sample invitation you can modify to host a healthy potluck dinner:

You're Invited to

A Healthy Potluck Dinner and Recipe Exchange!

Our goal is to bring people together who have an interest in eating healthier, trying new recipes, and having fun doing it.*

"Healthy" food is defined as vegetables, fruit, legumes, whole grains, nuts, and seeds. Recipes can be cooked or raw, from salads and soups to main courses and side dishes, and yes, desserts! (Please avoid using white flour, saturated fats, and added sugar.)

**Recipes can be emailed, bring one copy if you want it scanned to be sent out.*

Bring plenty of the food you are sharing, along with some containers to take some leftovers home (unless we eat it all).

When: 4th Sunday of the Month; September 23rd

Time: 6:00pm

Please RSVP by September 19th, and I will forward the address to you.

Who's Making Dinner Tonight?

How would it be to share the responsibility of cooking with your pre-teen or teenage kids, or other family members? They are capable of cooking once a week and can serve sandwiches, a salad, reheated leftovers, soup, or follow a recipe.

There are many benefits to assigning family members "cooking" nights.

1. It gives the person who generally cooks a night off and a chance to practice receiving.

2. It helps build confidence in the kitchen, a useful life skill.

3. It empowers the person cooking to decide what is going to be prepared; be it a simple sandwich, soup, or a 3-course meal.

4. It can bring a family together by sharing the responsibility of feeding each other.

With a little planning ahead, your family can take turns choosing and preparing nightly meals. And remember to give compliments to the chef!

Take Action:

There's no better time than NOW to decide to incorporate healthy eating into your lifestyle. If you haven't started yet, IT'S TIME to begin eating healthier!

Take action NOW to eat healthier with one or more options from the list below:

1. Refer to the numerous suggestions in this chapter of what healthier eating looks like. Make a list of foods that you want to eat. Then make a menu for breakfast, lunch, dinner, and snacks. Know ahead of time what you need to buy and prepare so that you can be successful.

2. Have healthy food choices with you. Pack your lunch and snacks.

3. Make extra servings when cooking. Cook up a large pot of soup, some extra vegetables, double a recipe, or set aside some time to make several different foods to get you through the week.

4. Host a Healthy Potluck Dinner. Select a date, contact some friends and family, and send out an invitation!

5. Delegate cooking to a family member. Let them pick out what will be prepared and served.

Notes

[1] The Pritikin Diet
https://www.webmd.com/diet/a-z/pritikin-diet

CHAPTER 16

Desserts, Holidays, and Travel

Most people indulge in food during the holiday season and while on vacation. In this chapter, you'll learn some ways to enjoy desserts, handle holiday eating and parties, and eat healthier while traveling.

There are lots of ways of approaching what you eat. Eating should be enjoyable, especially when you are making a change to improve your health. You don't have to give up anything, but you may want to consider some new ways of eating desserts in this chapter.

Healthy Eating and Desserts

You may be wondering if desserts, sweets, and treats fit into a healthy lifestyle. The short answer is yes, they can, just not daily. Here are some suggestions on how to enjoy something sweet:

1. Decide when, where, and with whom you will have your dessert. Make it a conscious decision.

2. Share one dessert. Ask for two spoons.

3. Whether alone or with others, enjoy a dessert by eating it with mindfulness.

4. Use the three-bite rule. Savor three bites or spoonful's and then remove it.

5. Use portion control and stick to one serving.

6. Have a dessert on special occasions like your birthday, anniversary, or a holiday.

7. Eat sweets out rather than at home where you may be tempted to overeat, especially if there is a large quantity or multiple servings.

8. Have a piece of fruit, melon, papaya, or berries when you are craving something sweet, or for dessert.

Holidays, Family Gatherings, and Celebrations

The months of November and December are when family and friends get together to celebrate holidays and attend parties. With food and drinks in abundance, not to mention candies, cookies, pies, and cakes, it's easy to let your healthy eating slide until January.

Minimize holiday weight gain by eating with mindfulness. When you deviate from your regular healthy eating, do it with awareness. Decide to indulge. Mindfully taste what you eat and drink. Savor each bite and sip. Eat slowly and put your fork down between bites. Check in with yourself after each bite and stop eating when that food item no longer tastes delicious, since the first few bites are generally the best tasting and most satisfying.

Serve yourself “taste-size portions” to sample rather than a plateful. Then go back for more of only the foods you found worthy. Remember that calories from holiday foods, drinks, desserts, and candies can add up much faster than you can burn them for energy.

Decide to eat a small meal, soup, salad, raw vegetables, or a piece of fruit before you go to a holiday event, dinner, or party, rather than arriving hungry. Then enjoy a sampling of foods while focusing on connecting with people rather than focusing on the food.

Healthy Eating Travel Tips

Whether you are traveling by car or by plane, heading to a campsite, taking a road trip or off to a hotel or resort destination, I’ve got some healthy eating tips for you.

Some of the best accommodation values are to rent a house, condo, or timeshare. All of these come with sizeable kitchens, making it easy to prepare healthy food while you are away.

If you’re driving to your destination, you can pack an ice chest with fruit, vegetables, and cooked lean meat, chicken, or salmon. The following precooked foods travel well: corn on the cob, brown rice, quinoa, lentils, and baked sweet potatoes. If you enjoy smoothies or protein shakes, it’s easy to bring a mini-blender and the ingredients. You can also bring canned food, tuna, corn, beans, and dry brown rice or quinoa and bottled water.

Consider what to bring based on the type of accommodations you will be staying at – can you cook or heat food? Do you have access to electricity and have refrigeration? (If you are crossing any borders into another state or country, be aware that they may have restrictions on produce and grains. The same applies to air travel into different countries.)

If you are staying at a hotel, you may have a small refrigerator and possibly a microwave oven. Camping will give you more options for cooking, but no electricity and no refrigeration. Keep in mind that an ice chest will not keep items as cold as a refrigerator. If you are flying to a destination where you will have a full kitchen, check out the options for grocery shopping by contacting the location where you will be staying or checking online.

If you are going to be preparing food while away, I recommend that you bring, or buy the following when you arrive: a roll of paper towels, a sponge, and some dishwashing soap. Not all places provide these items. You may also want to bring or buy storage containers or plastic bags for leftovers.

Travel Snack Bags

Regardless of where your destination is and if you are driving or flying, you can make a "Travel Snack Bag" for each person traveling. Some favorites to pack are whole wheat pretzels or whole grain crackers, a banana, apple, carrot sticks, red bell peppers, and almonds. You could also include a sandwich. Be aware that with the limitation of liquids on flights, this also applies to some foods, such as yogurt and hummus. If you are driving, everyone can have their own water. While traveling, each person can eat anything out of

their travel bag without having to ask or say they don't like any of the choices, especially if they helped pack their bag!
Happy Travels!

Take Action:

Life can be fun while eating healthy, enjoying celebrations or traveling! You will feel good and have a stronger immune system by eating well.

Try these suggestions the next time you have a celebration or travel:

1. Celebrating with a dessert on occasion is okay. Use some of the suggestions from, Healthy Eating and Desserts (on page 175). When you do have something sweet, be mindful and enjoy every bite of it!

2. Allow yourself to focus more on the company than on the food by not arriving hungry at a party or social event.

3. When traveling by airplane or by car, bring healthy food and snacks. When you get to your destination, if you are going to do some cooking, plan out a menu and go grocery shopping.

Part Six: Healthy Recipes

Very few people know that at the age of 26, I taught a lecture series at Pasadena City College on low-fat, low-cholesterol eating, and the following year taught cooking classes at a wellness center. Some of the recipes in this section are from those classes!

The following recipes are a great way to discover some new tastes. Experiment with different ingredients or seasonings. Once you find a recipe you enjoy, in its original form or modified, make a note of it so you can prepare it again.

Any recipe can be eaten at any time of day. Sometimes it's fun to have breakfast food for dinner and dinner food or leftovers for breakfast. Also, a side dish or appetizer can become a meal with a salad or soup.

I hope you, and your friends and family, like these recipes as much as mine do!

Start Your Day

Oatmeal Recipe Ideas

Prepare oatmeal according to the directions. Choose one or more from the following toppings and enjoy!

Fruit: 1/2 cup banana slices, chopped apple, fresh or frozen mixed berries or blueberries

Dried Fruit: 1 tablespoon raisins, cranberries, or chopped mangos or apricots

Nuts: 1 tablespoon chopped walnuts, almonds, or pecans

Seeds: 1 tablespoon chia seeds or 1 - 2 tablespoons ground flax seeds, or hemp seeds

Spices: 1 - 2 teaspoons cinnamon or 1/4 - 1/2 teaspoon pumpkin spice

Beverages: 1/2 cup of your choice; unsweetened almond, soy, rice, or coconut beverage, or non-fat or low-fat milk

Sample combinations:

Banana and walnuts

Cinnamon and chia seeds

Apples, pecans, and beverage of your choice

Blueberries, almonds, and beverage of your choice

Slow Cooker Apple Steel-Cut Oats

1-1/2 cups steel-cut oats

6 cups vanilla almond beverage, unsweetened

1 tablespoon cinnamon

1 tablespoon vanilla

2 apples, chopped

Place all of the ingredients into a slow cooker and stir. Cook on low for 8 hours, and you will have a healthy breakfast for the week.

Optional toppings:

1 tablespoon chopped walnuts, almonds, or pecans

1 tablespoon raisins, 1/2 sliced banana, or 1/2 cup berries.

For additional fiber, mix in 1 tablespoon of flax seeds or chia seeds before eating.

Cereals

Choose a high fiber (5 grams or more per serving), low sugar (5 - 7 grams or less per serving) breakfast cereal. Remember to look at the serving size. Add a beverage of your choice (unsweetened almond, rice, soy, or coconut beverage, or low-fat or non-fat milk), and fruit.

Yogurt and Add-Ins

Select a low sugar yogurt (less than 10 grams per serving). Greek yogurt tends to have less sugar and more protein. Plain yogurt will have less sugar, and you can add fruit, nuts, or spices.

Fruit: 1/2 cup fresh or frozen blueberries, raspberries, blackberries, diced peaches or nectarines, or banana.

Nuts: 1 tablespoon chopped walnuts, almonds, or pecans

Spices: 1 - 2 teaspoons cinnamon or 1/4 - 1/2 teaspoon pumpkin pie spice

Nut-Butter Sandwiches

2 slices whole grain bread or 1 thin whole wheat bun

2 tablespoons peanut butter, almond butter, or another nut butter

Sliced apple

Sliced banana

Toast bread, then spread one tablespoon of nut butter on each piece of bread and top with apple and banana slices.

Enjoy for breakfast, before a workout, for lunch, or as a snack.

Drinks

Nourishing Power Smoothie

1/2 cup water

1/2 banana (can be frozen)

1 peeled orange cut into sections

1/2 cup frozen blueberries

1 cup spinach

Place water in a blender, add banana, orange, blueberries, and spinach. Blend until smooth and enjoy!

Makes 2 servings.

Daryl's Very Green Smoothie

1/2 cucumber, chopped

1 cup of spinach

1/2 avocado

3 celery stalks, chopped

1/2 apple, chopped

1/2 cup of water

Place all ingredients in a blender and blend until smooth.

Makes 2 servings.

Super Green Smoothie

1 cup chopped cucumber

1 cup chopped celery

1 teaspoon fresh gingerroot, chopped

1 apple, chopped

1 cup spinach

1/3 cup fresh parsley

3 tablespoons lemon juice

Place all ingredients in a blender and blend until smooth.

Makes 2 servings.

Juicing Tips and Recipes

If you don't already have a juicer, look for one with a large opening to more easily fit fruit and vegetables without a lot of cutting.

It is best to drink freshly juiced produce at the time of juicing or within 48 hours.

Experiment with different combinations of vegetables and fruit. Use vegetables primarily and add a small amount of fruit to sweeten.

Here are some recipe combinations to get started:

Cucumber, celery, kale, apple

Cucumber, celery, kale, pear

Cucumber, celery, kale, pineapple

Beets, carrots, cucumber, parsley

Carrots, celery, cucumber

Carrots, celery, cucumber, ginger

Dips

Easy Homemade Hummus

2 large garlic cloves

1 can garbanzo beans (chickpeas) drained

2 tablespoons plain non-fat yogurt or water

2 tablespoons peanut butter or almond butter

2 tablespoons fresh lemon juice

1 teaspoon ground cumin

Salt and pepper (if desired)

Mince garlic in a food processor. Add remaining ingredients and blend, occasionally scraping down the sides of the work bowl. Continue blending until it reaches a smooth consistency. If too thick, add 1 - 2 tablespoons of water. If desired, season with salt and pepper. Transfer to a small bowl. Cover and store in the refrigerator. This recipe can be served cold or at room temperature.

Serving suggestions:

Enjoy with raw vegetables: carrots, celery, cucumbers, jicama, bell peppers (red, yellow, orange, or green), tomatoes, broccoli, or cauliflower.

Mix 2 tablespoons hummus with diced cucumbers and halved cherry tomatoes for a quick snack.

It's also great with toasted whole wheat pita bread.

Roasted Red Pepper Pesto Dip

2 large red bell peppers

1/2 cup walnuts, chopped

2 cloves garlic, minced

3 tablespoons olive oil

1/2 teaspoon salt

Preheat broiler. Cut peppers lengthwise in half and remove seeds. Place peppers cut side down on a foil-lined baking sheet. Broil for about 20 minutes, until charred. Cool, remove and discard skins. Cut peppers into wide strips.

Combine peppers, walnuts, garlic, oil, and salt in a food processor. Process until blended.

Makes about 1 cup.

Serve with toasted whole wheat pita bread or lightly steamed asparagus, broccoli, or other vegetables. It also goes well with pasta or chicken and can be used as a sandwich spread.

Soups

Michael's Vegetable Soup

1 tablespoon olive oil (or water)

1 cup chopped onion

1 cup diced carrots

1 can (28 ounces) tomato puree

4 - 5 cups vegetable or chicken broth, or water

1 can (15 ounces) cannellini (white kidney beans), undrained

1 can (15 ounces) corn, undrained

6 - 8 cups of various cut vegetables: zucchini, broccoli flowerets, cauliflower, asparagus, string beans, celery

2 teaspoons basil leaves, crushed

2 teaspoons oregano

1 teaspoon garlic powder

1 teaspoon onion powder

1 teaspoon salt (optional)

In a large soup pot, heat oil (or water) until hot. Add onion and carrots. Sauté for 3 minutes. Stir in tomato puree, broth or water, cannellini beans with liquid, corn with liquid, vegetables, and seasonings. Bring to a boil. Reduce heat and simmer covered for 45 minutes, stirring every 15 minutes until done.

Curry Lentil Soup

1 tablespoon water

1 onion, chopped

2 cloves garlic, minced

2 tablespoons curry powder

7 cups of water

1 cup carrots, chopped

2 cups fresh tomatoes, chopped or 1 can (14 - 16 ounces) tomatoes, diced

2 cups lentils, uncooked

In a large soup pot, heat 1 tablespoon of water, and the onion and garlic over medium heat, stirring occasionally, until the onion is translucent. Stir in the curry powder and continue stirring while it **cooks for one minute**. Add 7 cups of water, the carrots, tomatoes, and lentils. Bring to a boil, then cover and simmer over low heat for 45 minutes, until the lentils are cooked.

This makes a big pot full of soup that also freezes well.

Leftovers Soup

All you need is a leftover grain and some leftover vegetables. Add them to a broth of your choice.

2 cups broth (store bought or homemade)

1 cup cooked brown rice, quinoa, or whole grain pasta

1-1/2 cups chopped cooked leftover vegetables (broccoli, cauliflower, carrots, zucchini, bok choy, spinach, etc.)

In a saucepan, heat the broth. Add a cooked grain of choice and vegetables of choice. Heat thoroughly and enjoy.

Carrot Cauliflower Soup

2-1/2 cups vegetable broth (store bought or homemade)

1 cup onion, diced

1-1/2 pounds carrots, chopped into ½ inch pieces (about 5 - 7 large carrots)

3/4 pound baking potatoes, peeled and cut into ½ inch pieces

2 cups of water

1 pound cauliflower, in small florets (about 1-1/2 cups)

2 teaspoons rosemary, basil, or tarragon (fresh and chopped or dried)

Salt and pepper to taste, if desired

In a large soup pot, heat 1/4 cup vegetable broth. Add diced onion and simmer until onion is softened, about 5 minutes. Add carrots, potatoes, 2 more cups vegetable broth, and 2 cups of water. Bring to a boil. Cover and simmer for 5 minutes. Add cauliflower, cover and simmer until the vegetables are tender, 15 - 20 minutes.

Cool slightly, then puree in a blender or food processor until smooth. Return soup to the pot and stir in the seasoning of your choice. Reheat and if desired, add additional vegetable broth for a thinner consistency.

Celery Barley Soup

6 cups vegetable or chicken broth

1 cup onion, chopped

5 cups celery, sliced and divided

1/2 cup celery leaves, chopped

1 teaspoon thyme leaves, crushed

1 bay leaf

1/3 cup pearl barley

In a large soup pot, bring broth to a boil. Add onion, **3 cups celery,** celery leaves, thyme, and bay leaf. Bring to a boil and simmer covered for 30 minutes. **Remove bay leaf.** Puree soup in a blender in two batches. Return puree to the soup pot and bring to a boil. Add the barley and simmer covered until barley is almost tender, about 25 minutes. Add the remaining **2 cups celery.** Simmer covered until celery and barley are tender, about 5 minutes. Add salt and pepper if desired.

Black Bean Soup

1 cup onion, diced

2 cloves garlic, minced

1-1/4 cups vegetable broth (store bought or homemade)

2 (15-ounce) cans black beans (not drained)

1 (15-ounce) can diced tomatoes

1 cup baking potato, peeled and diced

1/2 teaspoon thyme

1/2 teaspoon cumin

Green onion, diced, for garnish

In a large soup pot, combine onion, garlic, and 1/4 cup vegetable broth. Bring to a simmer and cook for 3 - 5 minutes, until the onions are softened. Add 1 cup more of vegetable broth, black beans with the liquid, tomatoes, potatoes, thyme, and cumin. Bring to a simmer, cover and cook until the potatoes are tender, about 25 minutes. Add a little more broth to thin soup, if desired. Garnish with green onions.

Salads

Broccoli Cranberry Salad

4 cups broccoli florets, cut into small pieces

1/2 cup dried cranberries

1/4 cup minced red onion

1/3 cup olive oil

1/4 cup balsamic vinegar

Place broccoli, cranberries, and onion in a medium bowl. Next, mix the olive oil and vinegar and pour over the broccoli mixture. Toss well to coat with dressing. Cover and chill for at least one hour.

Sweet Potato Curry Bean Salad

2 cups cooked beans (a multi-bean blend of beans, lentils, and peas)

1 small sweet potato, baked in the skin and cut into diced pieces

1 tablespoon olive oil

1 clove garlic, minced

1/4 teaspoon curry powder

1/8 teaspoon salt (optional)

Prepare the dressing by mixing the olive oil, garlic, curry powder, and salt if desired. Place the beans in a bowl and stir in the dressing. Gently stir in the sweet potato pieces. Refrigerate for 2 hours or overnight.

Makes 4 servings.

Looks Cooked Raw Kale Salad

1 bunch kale

2 tablespoons lemon juice

1/4 teaspoon salt

1 teaspoon olive or walnut oil (if desired)

2 tablespoons chopped walnuts

Wash kale and remove the leaves from the thick stems. Place the kale leaves in a large bowl, drizzle with lemon juice and add salt. Massage the kale with your hands for several minutes. The kale will soften from the natural heat in your hands and the lemon juice and salt. Once it looks vibrant green and is softened, drizzle with oil, if desired, and top with chopped walnuts.

Other vegetables can be added to this salad: tomatoes, cucumber, shredded carrots, bell peppers, jicama, beets, etc.

Tomato Cucumber Salad

1 cup chopped tomato

1 cup diced cucumber

2 tablespoons hemp seeds

Combine tomatoes and cucumbers, then sprinkle with hemp seeds.

Makes 4 servings.

Black Bean Salad

2 cups black beans, drained and rinsed

1/2 cup yellow bell pepper, seeded and chopped

1/2 cup red bell pepper, seeded and chopped

1/2 cup cooked corn (fresh or canned)

1 tablespoon green onion, finely chopped

1 ripe avocado, diced

Dressing:

1 tablespoon olive oil

1 tablespoon fresh lime juice

1 clove garlic, minced

Optional: add salt and pepper to taste

Place beans, peppers, corn, and green onion in a bowl. Prepare the dressing by combining all the ingredients. Pour dressing over bean mixture and mix well. Cover and refrigerate for a few hours or overnight. Right before serving, add the avocado and mix gently, not to mash the avocado.

Serve as a side salad, on top of a green salad, with warm corn tortillas, or baked corn tortilla chips.

Beet Salad

3 large beets

Water

1/4 cup red onions, thinly sliced

1/4 cup white vinegar

1/4 cup olive oil

Preheat oven to 400 degrees. Wash the beets, cut off the tops, and place the beets in a covered baking dish with enough water to cover the bottom. Cook the beets until soft, about 60 - 75 minutes.

When the beets are cool enough to handle, remove the skin. It should peel off easily. Then slice the beets into thick bite-size pieces. Next, place the sliced beets into a container and add red onions, vinegar, and oil. Mix well and refrigerate covered for several hours or overnight. Serve cold as a side salad or on a green salad.

Cauliflower Salad

1 head cauliflower

1 bunch green onions

4 tablespoons olive oil

2 tablespoons lemon juice

1/2 cup cilantro, chopped

2 teaspoons onion powder

1/2 teaspoon sea salt

Prepare the dressing in a small bowl. Mix the olive oil, lemon juice, cilantro, onion powder, and salt. Set aside.

Chop the cauliflower and onions into small pieces. Place in a large bowl, add the dressing and mix well.

This recipe can be eaten immediately after preparing or can be refrigerated and served cold after marinating for several hours.

Main Dishes

Zucchini, Eggplant, Red Pepper Pasta

1 teaspoon olive oil

1 clove garlic, minced

2 medium zucchinis, cut into medium size pieces

1 small eggplant, cut into medium-size pieces

1 red bell pepper, cut into medium-size strips

1 package whole wheat or other whole grain pasta

Pasta sauce (optional)

Cook pasta according to instructions. While the pasta is cooking, heat olive oil in a large skillet. Cook the garlic until it starts to brown. Add the vegetables. Cook covered, occasionally stirring until the vegetables are soft. Add 1 - 2 tablespoons of water if the vegetables do not provide enough water during the cooking.

Serve the vegetables over the pasta and top with pasta sauce, if desired.

Tracie's Simple Pasta

1 package noodles (any shape), cooked

1 jar of marinara sauce

2 cups petite frozen peas

Combine cooked noodles, sauce, and peas in a large pot. Heat and serve.

Healthy Fish Tacos

2 pieces of Mahi Mahi or other white fish

Olive oil, to drizzle on fish

Cumin, a sprinkle

1 lime

1 red bell pepper, sliced into quarters

4 corn tortillas, warmed on the grill, barbecue, or stove

Lettuce and cilantro, chopped

Drizzle fish with olive oil, then sprinkle with cumin. Squeeze lime juice on the fish and set aside for 15 minutes.

Grill the fish and red pepper on an indoor grill or outdoor barbecue until done. Slice the fish, and red peppers into strips. Serve on top of warm corn tortillas and top with lettuce and cilantro.

Makes 2 servings.

Optional serving ideas: top tacos with sliced avocado and salsa.

Serve with a side or two from these: jicama, carrots, mango, watermelon, brown rice, quinoa, whole pinto beans or black beans.

Lentils with Broccoli and Pasta Sauce

1 cup precooked lentils, per serving

3/4 cup broccoli, steamed, per serving

Pasta sauce

Heat lentils and broccoli and top with sauce and enjoy!

Spaghetti Squash and Caramelized Onions

1 spaghetti squash

2 - 4 tablespoons olive oil

2 onions, chopped

Salt (optional)

Cut spaghetti squash in half lengthwise and scoop out seeds. Bake cut side down on a baking pan at 350 degrees for 45 minutes. Rotate pan and cook an additional 30 minutes or until skin is tender. While the squash is cooking, place the olive oil and onions in a frying pan and cook, frequently stirring, until browned. Season with salt, if desired.

Once the squash is cool enough to handle, use a fork to scrape out the strands of squash. Gently fold in the caramelized onions. Season with salt if desired.

Makes 4 servings.

Rice, Beans, and Tomato

Precooked brown rice and a can of refried beans make this single-serving recipe quick and easy!

1/2 cup vegetarian refried beans (canned or homemade)

1/2 cup brown rice, cooked

1 tomato, diced

Oregano

1 tablespoon green onion, sliced

Heat refried beans and rice individually, then combine them. Fold in the diced tomato. Top with a sprinkle of oregano and sliced green onion.

Makes 2 servings.

Enjoy with a salad for a meal or as a side dish with chicken, fish, or lean meat and a serving or two of vegetables.

White Bean Lettuce Wrap

1 (15 oz.) can white beans, drained and slightly mashed

1/4 cup red onion, finely chopped

1/2 cup celery, diced into small pieces

Dressing:

1 tablespoon olive oil

3 tablespoons lemon juice or juice of one lemon

1/4 teaspoon dill

Salt and pepper to taste (optional)

4 whole leaves of romaine lettuce

Place mashed beans into a bowl. Add red onion and celery. Prepare the dressing of olive oil, lemon juice, dill, salt, and pepper, if desired. Then mix the dressing into the bean mixture. Spoon the bean mixture onto the middle of 4 whole lettuce leaves, wrap and enjoy.

Makes 4 servings.

Vegetarian Multi-Bean Chili

If using dried beans, plan on soaking the beans overnight and allow about two hours to cook the beans. I use a blend of beans that also included lentils and peas. The simple way is to use precooked or canned beans.

1/4 cup olive oil

1 large onion, chopped

1 red bell pepper, diced

6 cloves garlic, minced

1-1/2 tablespoon chili powder

1-1/2 teaspoons dried oregano

1-1/2 teaspoons ground cumin

1 teaspoon salt

1-1/2 cups water

6 cups cooked beans

1 (14.5 oz.) can diced tomatoes

Heat oil in a large soup pot. Add onion, red bell pepper, and garlic. Sauté until the vegetables are soft. Add the chili powder, oregano, cumin, and salt. Stir over heat for 2 minutes. Stir in the water, cooked beans, and tomatoes. Bring to a boil, reduce heat and simmer, occasionally stirring, until the chili thickens and the flavors blend, about 30 minutes.

Makes 8 - 10 servings.

Vegetable Stir-Fry

Any combination of vegetables will work in this recipe.

2 teaspoons garlic, fresh and minced

1/2 - 1 teaspoon ginger, fresh and chopped

1/4 - 1/2 cup vegetable broth

4 - 5 cups vegetables cut into small pieces (so they will cook quickly). Choose your vegetables from the following: (About 5 different ones make a good stir-fry, about 1 cup of each.) Asparagus, snow peas, carrots, broccoli, cauliflower, cabbage, bok choy, bell peppers, mushrooms, zucchini, onions.

Optional: 1-1/2 cups bean sprouts (fresh), 1 can bamboo shoots, or 1 can water chestnuts

In a large skillet or wok, simmer the garlic and ginger in 1/4 cup vegetable broth for 3 minutes. Add 4 - 5 cups vegetables. Cook over moderately high heat, frequently stirring until vegetables begin to soften. Continue to cook until vegetables are tender-crisp, about 5 minutes. Add bean sprouts, bamboo shoots, and water chestnuts, if using, and cook until hot.

Serve over brown rice.

Tostadas with Baked Tortillas

6 corn tortillas

1 can vegetarian refried beans

Lettuce, shredded

1 large or 2 small avocados, sliced

2 tomatoes, sliced

Bake tortillas at 300 degrees. Turn after 10 minutes, check after another 5 minutes and turn again. Bake until crisp and just browned, about 20 minutes total time.

Heat beans and spread about 1/4 cup on each baked tortilla. Top with lettuce, tomato, and avocado. Serve with a side of jicama.

Makes 6 tostadas.

Zucchini Pasta

1 tablespoon olive oil

5 - 7 zucchini, (spiralized in a turning slicer, to look like long spaghetti noodles or shredded)

2 cloves garlic, minced

1/4 teaspoon oregano

White beans (15-ounce can), drained

Optional: pasta sauce or tomato sauce

Heat oil in a large frying pan. Add zucchini and cook covered, frequently checking, until it becomes a bit soft, like cooked noodles. Stir in garlic and oregano, then the beans. Cook until heated. Depending on the water content of the zucchini, you may already have a natural "sauce." The cooked zucchini can be topped with pasta sauce or tomato sauce.

Sides

Roasted Cauliflower

Wait! Don't skip this recipe! If you are not a fan of cauliflower, don't leave! Cauliflower was never my favorite until I roasted it. Roasting brings out the sweetness. The taste is so delicious that it's hard to believe that it's the same food as when it is steamed. Try it, and it may become one of your favorites too!

1 medium head cauliflower (2-1/2 to 3 pounds), cut into small pieces

2 tablespoons extra-virgin olive oil

1/4 teaspoon salt

Preheat oven to 450°F. Coat cauliflower with oil in a large bowl. Line a large, 1-inch deep baking pan with parchment paper. Place the cauliflower on the pan in a single layer and sprinkle with salt. Roast the cauliflower, turning it over occasionally, until tender and golden brown, 25 to 35 minutes.

Zucchini Rice Bake

1 cup cooked brown rice

1 tablespoon olive oil

1 onion, diced

4 medium zucchinis, diced

Oregano, thyme, or rosemary

Optional: pasta sauce or tomato sauce

Sauté the onion in olive oil until soft, add zucchini and 1/4 to 1/2 cup water. Cook until zucchini is done, depending on your desired texture. Mix in cooked brown rice. Place in a baking pan and sprinkle with seasoning of choice. Top with sauce, if desired. Bake covered at 350 degrees for 40 minutes. Enjoy as a side dish or with a salad.

Steamed Vegetable Medley

1 onion, chopped

1 red bell pepper, cut into bite-size pieces

1 - 2 zucchini, sliced

1/2 bunch asparagus, cut into 1-inch pieces

1 bunch broccoli, cut into small pieces

1/4 head cauliflower, cut into bite-size pieces

1 handful green beans, cut into 1-inch pieces

In a large pot, place a steamer basket and fill with water to the top of the basket. If you don't have a steamer basket, fill the pot with 3 inches of water. Add all the vegetables and cook covered (occasionally stirring if you aren't using a steamer basket), until the vegetables begin to soften.

Serve as a side dish or over whole wheat pasta or brown rice. Top with sauce if desired.

Quinoa, Cranberries, and Green Onions

3 cups quinoa, cooked

1/4 cup dried cranberries

2 tablespoons sliced green onions

While quinoa is warm, stir in dried cranberries and green onions. Serve warm or cold.

Makes 6 servings.

Quinoa, Caramelized Onions, and Broccoli

1 onion, chopped

1 tablespoon olive oil

2 cups steamed broccoli or other precooked vegetables cut into small pieces

2 cups cooked quinoa

In a large frying pan, cook the onions in olive oil until darkly browned. The more browned the onions, the sweeter they will taste. Add the cooked broccoli or other vegetables to the onions and mix well. Continue to cook until heated. Gently mix in the cooked quinoa, cook until heated.

Serve warm as a side dish or cold on a salad.

Makes 4 servings.

Broccoli with Cooked Fresh Tomatoes

1 teaspoon olive oil

1 clove garlic, chopped

2 fresh tomatoes, diced

1 cup broccoli, steamed (precooked)

Salt and oregano or basil to taste

Heat oil in a medium pan. Cook garlic until just starting to brown. Stir in tomatoes and sauté until they are softened. Season with salt and oregano or basil to taste. Add broccoli and stir until mixed well.

Makes 2 servings.

Eat as a side dish or serve over brown rice or whole grain pasta. For a heartier meal, add in cooked lentils, white beans, or quinoa.
This recipe can also be served cold or added to a salad.

Delicious Greens with Garlic

2 cups or more of greens (spinach, kale, beet greens, chard), washed, removed from thick stems, and torn into pieces

1/2 tsp. olive oil

2 cloves garlic, finely chopped

Salt and pepper, to taste if desired

Lemon juice

Heat the oil, then add the greens and garlic. Cook covered, turning frequently, and remove from heat when wilted. Season with salt and pepper if desired, and a squeeze of lemon.

Cauliflower Fried Rice

1 cauliflower "riced," see below how to "rice" cauliflower or use store bought (about 3 cups)

1/4 cup chopped red onion

1/4 cup chopped carrot

1/2 red bell pepper, chopped

1/2 cup frozen peas

1 cup chopped bok choy

2 tablespoons olive oil

Water

How to "rice" cauliflower: Cut cauliflower from its thick stem and into medium size pieces. Grate into rice in a food processor in two batches, using the metal blade, not a grating disc.

Heat olive oil in a large frying pan and add grated cauliflower. Cook on medium heat, covered, for 4 minutes, then stir and add 1/3 cup water. Cook covered for 4 more minutes. Add more water if necessary, to prevent sticking. Stir in the remaining vegetables and cook covered until they begin to soften, about 4 more minutes.

Eggplant and Greens

1 eggplant, cubed

2 teaspoons olive oil (divided)

Water

1/8 teaspoon oregano

Salt, to taste if desired

1 bunch greens (beet greens, spinach, kale, or collard greens), washed and removed from any thick stems. Tear extra large pieces into smaller ones.

Coat a large frying pan with 1 teaspoon of olive oil. Add the eggplant cubes and cook for 1 minute, add 1/2 cup water, oregano, and salt, if desired, and stir. Sauté eggplant covered, stirring frequently. Add more water if necessary. Cook until eggplant softens. Remove cooked eggplant from the pan and set aside. Using the same frying pan, place 1 teaspoon olive oil and greens, sprinkle with oregano and salt, if desired, and sauté until wilted. Place the greens on a serving dish and top with eggplant or mix them together.

Makes 2 - 4 servings.

Stuffed Acorn Squash

2 acorn squash

1 cup quinoa (uncooked)

2 cups water or vegetable broth

1 teaspoon olive oil

1 teaspoon pumpkin spice

1/4 teaspoon turmeric

1/4 cup red onion, diced

2 tablespoons cranberries, dried

Cut the squash in half, remove seeds, and bake at 400 degrees, cut side down on a lined baking sheet until soft, about 30 - 40 minutes. While the squash is cooking, prepare the filling. Rinse the quinoa and place in a medium saucepan with the remaining ingredients. Bring to a boil, then reduce the heat and simmer, covered, for 15 minutes. Let sit covered for an additional 5 - 10 minutes. Fluff with a fork.

When the squash is done, stuff both halves with the quinoa filling and sprinkle with additional pumpkin spice.

Makes 4 servings.

Roasted Butternut Squash

1 butternut squash, peeled and cubed

Olive oil

Pinch of nutmeg

1/4 teaspoon cinnamon

1/4 teaspoon dried garlic or garlic powder

Place cubed squash in a bowl, lightly drizzle with olive oil, add remaining ingredients, and mix well. Spread on a parchment paper, or a foil-lined baking sheet and bake at 400 degrees for 30 minutes, turning after 15 minutes. Place under the broiler for 5 - 10 minutes to brown. Check frequently.

Asparagus, Red Peppers and Onions

1 bunch asparagus, washed and ends trimmed

1 or 2 red bell peppers, sliced into strips

1 or 2 onions, sliced

Olive oil

Onion or garlic powder or salt (optional)

Lightly coat vegetables with olive oil and spread in a single layer on two baking sheets lined with parchment paper or foil. Sprinkle with seasonings if desired. Cook at 425 degrees for 20 minutes, turn over with a spatula and cook for an additional 20 minutes or until the vegetables are tender and browned on the edges.

Sweets

Refreshing Raspberry Fruit Salad

1 10 oz. package of unsweetened frozen raspberries

3 grapefruits, peeled, sectioned, and sliced into bite-size pieces

2 ripe bananas, thinly sliced

Place frozen raspberries in a medium bowl. Add the grapefruit pieces and mix well. Just before serving, add the sliced bananas.

Yummy Yam Pudding

4 medium-size yams

1 acorn squash, cut in half and seeded

1/4 teaspoon cinnamon

Preheat oven to 400 degrees. Bake yams and squash together by placing the yams on the top oven rack with foil below to catch any dripping, and the squash, cut side down, on a foil or parchment paper-lined baking sheet. Bake until both are soft (test by inserting a knife), about one hour, turning the yams after 30 minutes.

When cooled enough to handle, peel the yams and scrape the squash from the outer shell. Place in a large bowl, add the cinnamon. Using a hand mixer, beat until smooth. Enjoy warm or cold.

Makes 6 servings.

Pumpkin-Banana Almond Cookies

1 cup banana puree (2 medium bananas mashed well)

1 teaspoon vanilla

1 teaspoon pumpkin pie spice

1/4 cup chopped almonds

1 1/2 cup uncooked oatmeal

Pour banana puree into a bowl. Add vanilla and pumpkin pie spice and stir. Add the almonds and oatmeal and mix well. Drop by tablespoonsful onto a cookie sheet lined with non-stick foil or parchment paper. Bake at 375 degrees for 20 minutes.

Recipe Index

Salads

Main Dishes

Sides

Sweets

Acknowledgments

Tired and Hungry No More – Not Your Ordinary Guide to Reclaiming Your Health and Happiness, came together to be a much richer book because of the support and a collaboration of many people. I'd first like to extend a BIG thank you to Vicki Dello Joio who encouraged me to be vulnerable and share more of me in the book.

Another BIG thank you goes to my husband Michael, who has been supportive of me living my life in ways that are satisfying to me, especially as I've spent hours and hours writing and editing this book.

Everyone who is in my Tapped In Community, is or was a client, or participated in the first Tired and Hungry No More Workshop, helped make this a better book! It's because of our work together that I have been able to put the pieces together for others to benefit. Thank you for being who you are and allowing me to grow and learn from our work together!

Maura McCarley Torkildson, Bettyanne Green and Sharon Esposito carefully read each page of my manuscript and enriched this book with their feedback and suggestions. I am grateful for your contributions!

Lastly, thanks to Vicki Dello Joio and Suzanne Waligore for coming up with the title and subtitle.

PHYLLIS GINSBERG

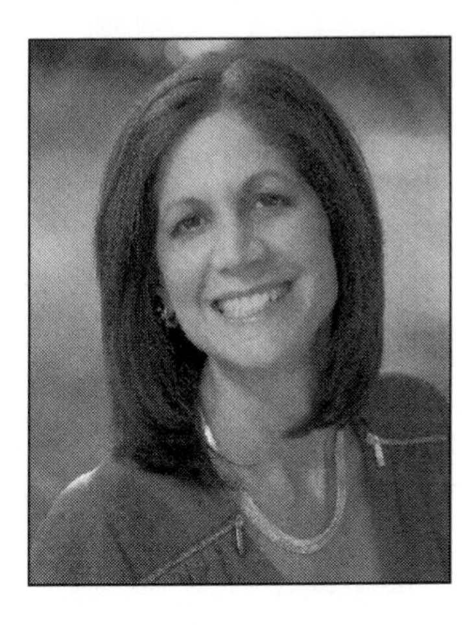

Phyllis Ginsberg is the creator of the Tapped In Community. She has helped change the lives of over 1,000 people with her ability to get to the heart of the matter quickly. Phyllis has three decades of experience as a Marriage and Family Therapist, expertise in Positive Psychology, Brain Research, and EFT Tapping.

Phyllis served on the task force committee for the American Heart Association and was a volunteer with the American Stroke Association, training adults to complete their first half marathon. She conducts workshops for the Cancer Support Community of the San Francisco Bay Area and was selected as a speaker for the American Cancer Society for Northern California 2017.

Phyllis and her husband live in the San Francisco Bay Area where she has a private practice. For more information about Phyllis' work, visit www.phyllisginsberg.com.

Also by Phyllis Ginsberg

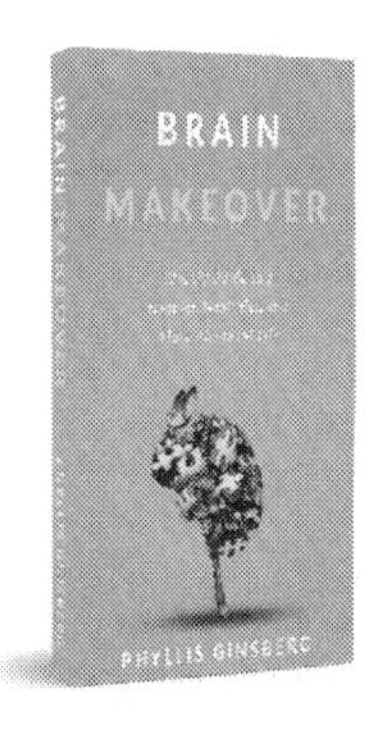

If you enjoyed *Tired and Hungry No More*, you'll want to read *Brain Makeover – A Weekly Guide to a Happier, Healthier and More Abundant Life.*

Brain Makeover is based on Positive Psychology and brain research for the most up to date personal development tools to experience a better understanding of how your, thoughts affect your health and happiness.

Practical and easy to follow messages will inspire you to take the steps necessary to have the life you deeply desire. Each week you will be guided to think about or do something that will have you on your way to building new neural pathways and lasting changes for a happier, healthier and more abundant life!

For more about Phyllis' work and to receive her valuable newsletter, visit www.phyllisginsberg.com.

Made in the USA
Middletown, DE
06 December 2019

80138458R00135